Sex & Fertility
Natural Solutions

Sex & Fertility
Natural Solutions

Linda Woolven <small>(M.H., C.Ac.)</small> **& Ted Snider**

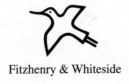

Fitzhenry & Whiteside

Published in Canada by Fitzhenry & Whiteside, 195 Allstate Parkway, Markham, Ontario L3R 4T8
Published in the United States by Fitzhenry & Whiteside, 311 Washington Street, Brighton,
Massachusetts 02135

10 9 8 7 6 5 4 3 2 1

Library and Archives Canada Cataloguing in Publication
Woolven, Linda
Sex & fertility : natural solutions / Linda Woolven & Ted Snider.
Includes index.
ISBN 978-1-55455-128-6
1. Reproductive health--Popular works. 2. Infertility--Alternative treatment--Popular works.
3. Sexual health--Popular works. 4. Sexual disorders--Alternative treatment--Popular works. 5.
Naturopathy-- Popular works. I. Snider, Ted II. Title. III. Title: Sex and fertility.
RG133.W66 2011   613.9   C2011-907145-2

Publisher Cataloging-in-Publication Data (U.S)
Woolven, Linda.
Sex & fertility : natural solutions / Linda Woolven ; Ted Snider.
[ ] p. : ill. ; cm.
Includes index.
Summary: A collection of natural medicinal solutions to infertility and reproductive health. Combin-
ing tradition, modern and natural medicine, this book examines ancient aphrodisiacs, and answers
questions about male and female infertility and libido, erectile dysfunction, premature ejaculation,
vaginal dryness, postpartum depression, and low libido after birth.
ISBN: 978-1-55455-128-6 (pbk.)
1. Infertility--Alternative treatment--Popular works. 2. Reproductive health--Popular works. 3.
Sexual health--Popular works. I. Snider, Ted. II. Sex and fertility. III. Title.
613.9 dc23 RG133.W664 2012

Fitzhenry & Whiteside acknowledges with thanks the Canada Council for the Arts and the Ontario
Arts Council for their support of our publishing program. We acknowledge the financial support of
the Government of Canada through the Canada Book Fund (CBF) for our publishing activities.

 Canada Council Conseil des Arts
for the Arts du Canada 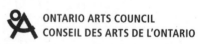 **ONTARIO ARTS COUNCIL**
CONSEIL DES ARTS DE L'ONTARIO

Design by Daniel Choi
Cover image courtesy of GettyImages
Printed in Canada by Friesens

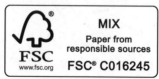

MIX
Paper from
responsible sources
FSC **FSC® C016245**
www.fsc.org

"To the hope and happiness that this book will bring."

About the Authors

Linda Woolven (M.H., C.Ac.) is a master herbalist and acupuncturist, and a certified solution-focused counselor practicing in Toronto. Linda Woolven and Ted Snider are authors of *The Family Naturopathic Encyclopedia*, *Healthy Herbs*, and *The Vegetarian Passport Cookbook*.

Praise for *Sex & Fertility*

This book is packed full of effective natural approaches to deal with problems common to both men and women.

—Michael T. Murray, N.D., co-author of *Encyclopedia of Natural Medicine*

A well-documented and enjoyable resource book on alternative approaches to aphrodisiacs, erectile dysfunction and infertility. Full of fun lore and useful information. Lay readers and professionals can, like me, enjoy and learn from this book. Fun reading; good information.

—James A. Duke, USDA (ret.), author of *The Green Pharmacy Guide to Healing Foods*
(Rodale Press, 2009)

I love this book! It's well researched, comprehensive and a delight to read. Filled with great information, wonderful herbal stories and sound advice, *Sex & Fertility* provides information one needs to know to enhance one's sexual energy naturally. It also provides excellent solutions for many of the daunting reproductive problems that are currently on the rise.

—Rosemary Gladstar, Herbalist and Author

Contents

introduction

HOLISTIC SOLUTIONS FOR FERTILITY, VIRILITY, AND LIBIDO: HEALTHY SEX

Y ou can have healthy, happy sex throughout your life and all throughout your senior years—you just need to know how. And this book
will tell you, whether you are male or female.

This book will tell you how to naturally improve infertility, libido, virility,
erectile dysfunction, and other problems that can interfere with sex and reproduction.

A verdict of infertility no longer has to be a life sentence against creating new
life. And this book will tell you why.

Sex & Fertility will pull back the curtains on nature's secrets for maintaining
and re-arousing virility and fertility. For most frustrated couples, a doctor's
diagnosis of infertility represents the end of their natural quest for children
and the beginning of their surrender to their fate or of their refuge in an im-
personal world of expensive and often ineffective medications that may have
undesirable side effects and often don't even work.

What most couples don't know is that there is a host of simple lifestyle factors that are totally in our control that can affect our fertility and that altering them can reawaken it. By changing those lifestyle factors, we can stay on the path to natural pregnancy. And when lifestyle changes are not enough, there are all kinds of safe, natural herbal and vitamin alternatives to those unnatural medical pills.

More than anything lately, I see couples in my clinic who are having trouble conceiving and who have tried all of the various procedures that conventional medicine has to offer, to no avail. Getting pregnant is not supposed to be this complicated.

Infertility is technically defined as the inability to conceive after one year of unprotected intercourse. It is possible, though, to have a baby after a year, and it is likely to become frustrating and feel like infertility long before a year. Fixing this frustrating problem is usually a team effort: both the male and the female have to make changes and try new things. This is both because the causes are equally likely to lie in either—40% of the time the woman's health is at issue, 40% of the time it's the man's, and 20% of the time it's both of you—and because going through it together is emotionally supporting.

There are many factors in our modern lifestyle that threaten fertility. It wasn't always this way. In our grandparents' and great-grandparents' time, we were so fertile that not having babies was the challenge. Now, having babies is such a challenge, fertility clinics—an inconceivable concept only a generation ago—are proliferating faster than we are. Why is this happening? How have our world and our lifestyle changed between the fertile generations and now?

There are a variety of reasons, some of which have to do with the emphasis people are placing on suddenly trying to get pregnant when *they* want to as opposed to the old days when people just got pregnant as a matter of course. It was not like it is now. There was no "Okay, it's time to try." The old, natural way created a lot less pressure—watching carefully to see if it worked, to see if I'm pregnant—and a lot less stress. Which leads to the first reason that I find couples have trouble getting pregnant. Stress. The more anxious you are, the harder it is to get pregnant. To women, this is not surprising: remember other times in your life when you were really stressed, and how that could alter your cycle? Well, it is doing the same thing now and making it hard to conceive. In the chapter on female infertility, you'll see not only why, but scientific proof that ending the stress might end the infertility. And though men are less likely to talk about stress, they are no less likely to suffer from it. In the chapters on male impotence and infertility, you'll see that stress is a cause of problems in men, too. Several of the herbs that help men double as calming herbs that provide support in times of stress. And, as you'll see in the next chapter, many of those traditional and magical aphrodisiacs may actually work by smoothing our nerves and stress.

Today, we are also eating more and more bad foods that make getting pregnant difficult. Our grandparents and great-grandparents didn't do that. Ours is a culture of fast food, too many animal products, and lots of sugar, caffeine, and refined, chemical-laced, nutrient-depleted, empty foods. Combined with our overstressed, unbalanced lives, these sound like strange times in which to bring a baby into the world. Our culture has moved away from the natural, whole-food diet that we evolved to thrive on. No wonder infertility rates are on the rise.

None of this dietary advice needs to be confusing or hard to sort out. *Sex & Fertility* will clearly lead you through the maze of modern research and set you on the simple and satisfying path of food for fertility. We will reveal the groundbreaking research that proves that diet is as important for female fertility as it is for heart health, diabetes, or any other matter of health, and that it is no less crucial for men.

Today we are also exercising less, using hot tubs, saunas, and wearing non-breathable fabrics. What do fabrics and saunas have to do with it? You'll be surprised to see in the chapter on male infertility that, for some men who want to be fathers, fabrics and saunas are the final blow. And exercising less may sound strange with a gym on every corner, but the truth is that we exercise either less than previous generations or excessively; and, as you'll see in the chapters on male and female fertility and erectile dysfunction, both can cause problems. Most of us don't get the same amount of natural exercise that we would have a couple of generations ago. Work was more labour intensive, both on the job and around the house; we had fewer machines to do the work for us, and we were not always on the computer or in front of the TV.

In addition to diet and exercise, other lifestyle and environmental factors have also changed between the fertile generations and now. Our world is newly full of chemicals and food additives. It is full of estrogen-containing pills, pesticides, and plastics. Can you imagine what that does to your reproductive system? And today we are also radiated and medicated—medicated on drugs that can sink your libido and destroy your chances of having a baby—and of having an erection!

And for those times when diet, lifestyle, and environmental solutions are not enough, *Sex & Fertility* will also make available to you both the most modern science and the most ancient traditions of herbs, vitamins, and nutrients for fertility, libido, and virility. You will be amazed as the medical myth that there is no science behind herbs and vitamins explodes before your eyes with an array of research on natural supplements for female infertility and male infertility and erectile dysfunction. Every chapter throughout *Sex & Fertility* is bursting with exciting studies, traditions, and clinical cases that show you how to solve your problem and enhance your fertility and virility with herbs, vitamins, and nutrients.

Though dietary and lifestyle lists of what to avoid when you are trying to have a baby may seem daunting, fertility and sexuality are not just about what you don't do, they are also about what you *do* do. And this book will help you to do that, too! *Sex & Fertility* is bursting with information on how to stoke libido and keep up everything else that you need to keep up! We will introduce you to the sometimes hilarious and mysterious folkloric world of aphrodisiacs and potions that at one time or another were believed to help you perform. And we will amaze you with how often these ancient and medieval potions are resurrected and vindicated by modern science. The secret aphrodisiac wisdom of the ancients will be uncovered and made available to you!

Sex & Fertility will answer all your reproductive-health questions, not only about fertility, libido, and virility, but also about making sex easy and satisfying, from problems almost everyone experiences at some time, such as premature ejaculation or vaginal dryness, to recovering from postpartum depression and low libido after birth, to enriching your self-image and sexuality after menopause. It will also talk about the relationship of urinary tract infections, candida, and enlarged prostate to sex and fertility.

And, because sex and having a baby are supposed to be enjoyable, we have tried to make this book enjoyable, too. So, while you are learning all the latest in the field of natural and all the oldest of the wisdom of tradition, have fun reading all the amusing tales and funny facts that we have interspersed throughout this book.

Be healthy, be happy, and be bursting with life!

Part I

Love Potions: The History of Using Nature
to Boost Fertility and Sexuality

Chapter One

FOLKLORE, POTIONS, AND APHRODISIACS

Who hasn't at some time in life felt unrequited love, or at least desire, and wished there was some magic herb that would make the object of our affection love or, at the very least, desire us back? It is often the stuff of good literature. Well, look at the long list of herbs below—perhaps your wish is about to be granted! But the question is how to get the herb to make the person favour only you? This is one dilemma that we still have not found an answer to, but perhaps desire is the first step, and the rest will follow.

Every culture has a wide variety of herbs and other remedies that are supposed to make you more virile and more fertile. While some may seem truly outrageous, some are actually proven by science to work, and to work as well or better than the sometimes rather dangerous drugs.

The sheer number of herbs that have been believed to possess aphrodisiac powers suggests that people everywhere in every age have sought herbal help for fertility and reproductive power. When we turned to Walter Lewis and Memory Elvin-Lewis's authoritative textbook on medicinal plants, we were surprised to find a chart spreading over several pages and listing sixty-eight herbs that have been used as aphrodisiacs[1]. And that, it turned out, was nothing. When we contacted James Duke, an ethnobotanist, and one of the world's leading experts on herbs, who has traveled the world gathering information on how they are used in different cultures, he was so generous as to give us access to his database of herbs that have been used as folkloric aphrodisiacs—a database that contained 321 aphrodisiac herbs! There is an ancient and intimate relationship between man and nature in the quest for enhanced sexual power.

SOME COMMON PLANTS USED TRADITIONALLY AS APHRODISIACS

Anise	Gotu kola
Asparagus	Hibiscus
Apricot	Kava kava
Basil	Magnolia
Bitter melon	Mandrake
Burdock	Marijuana
Cardamom	Morning glory
Cayenne	Mugwort
Celery	Muira puama
Chastetree berry	Mullein
Chocolate	Myrrh
Codonopsis	Nettle
Coriander	Nutmeg
Cotton	Onion
Damiana	Parsley
Dong quai	Passionflower
Echinacea angustifolia	Peppermint
Fava beans	Plantain
Fenugreek	Poppy seed
Ginger	Rhodiola rosea
Ginseng	Saffron
Goji berry (wolf berry)	Sage

Sarsaparilla	Truffles (mushroom)
Saw palmetto berry	Vanilla
Summer savory	Vervain
Sunflower	Watercress
Tribulus	Yohimbe

Frequently, on our travels, we have heard of a local remedy that is reputed—and much consumed—to increase fertility and vigour. And, in fact, when we get home and look into the stories, there is usually at least some truth to them.

DO APHRODISIACS REALLY WORK?

As you will see in the following chapters, some herbs and nutrients really do help with fertility, sexual function, and performance. But can some herbs and foods really flame desire and fire your passion? Are any of the legendary aphrodisiacs really for real? According to modern science, it certainly seems so.

For many, probably the majority, of aphrodisiac herbs, the effect, though perhaps no less real, is more indirect. Many aphrodisiac herbs work not so much by adding desire, but by removing impediments to desire. Those impediments may be different for different people. Some people need to relax and eliminate the frayed nerves, stress, and anxiety that are impeding desire. Many traditional aphrodisiac herbs—such as passionflower, kava kava, vervain, and ginseng—may work in part by soothing our nerves and calming our stress. Some people are just too exhausted and burnt out to burn with a higher flame. And some traditional aphrodisiacs—such as chocolate, cayenne, ginseng, ginger, and cinnamon—may work in part by stimulating or boosting energy.

Throughout this chapter on folkloric potions and aphrodisiacs, we will place an asterisk[*] beside those herbs and foods that have traditionally been esteemed as powerful aphrodisiacs and that will have their scientific vindication fully discussed in later chapters.

Hard Wine

One local remedy in particular comes to mind. It is a herb called horny goat weed. The name says it all. Even better, it comes in a form that is called hard wine—another great name. On a trip to Tobago, we were invited to a street party of dancing and celebrating. It was dark and late. A local man decided to teach Linda some of the local dances. Only, after a while, she realized that he was a little too eager and, as the wine's name suggests, already in position. We disengaged and, with the other celebrants, watched the night unfold.

The next day at the stunning local beach, the man, whose name turns out to be Jungle, and his friend Hollis, explain to us the secret that allows them to drink this stuff all day: "And you don't get drunk doing it," he claims, while we're thinking he's clearly getting drunker and drunker as he speaks. He's not as drunk as we would be if we drank what he was drinking, but, nevertheless, he's ready to go again. The hard wine is clearly working.

So what is in this remarkable stuff? Most people would be less able to rise to the occasion after so much to drink.

Horny goat weed. Hard wine combines horny goat weed with eleuthero* (formerly known as Siberian ginseng) and a mysterious tree bark called bois bandé, soaked in a red fruit wine. Does it really work? Hollis, a really great guy whose mother is a herbalist, says it does. His partner says if you want to know the truth, don't ask the husbands, ask the wives.

"Does it really work?" we ask Hollis's partner.

"Oh yeah!" she smiles.

But the story gets better. A few days later, the night before we leave, some friends we'd met on the island decided unexpectedly to come to our cottage. Linda was in the bathroom, getting ready for bed. Everything was packed but the unopened bottle of hard wine—purely market research for this book and for photographs, honest! But coming in and finding Linda running for cover and the unopened bottle of hard wine lying on the bed, they ask, "Have we come at a bad time?" They know which book we're currently researching and writing and they know about hard wine.

We got a good laugh out of that one. And we had a good night's sleep, too. We were not intending to try the wine that night.

But horny goat weed does have a tradition of increasing virility and fertility. So can it? And eleuthero has both a long tradition and modern science behind it. Bois bandé is more of a mystery. A major ingredient in the hard wine and the one everybody talked about, it is a herb we have been able to find virtually nothing reliable on. However, we did find an interview with healers from Trinidad and Tobago in which bois bandé (*Richeria grandis*) came up as a treatment for erectile dysfunction, so who knows? And what of the classically named horny goat weed? Let's look.

Horny Goat Weed

This herb has been used in China for over a thousand years, where it is known as *yin yang huo*, which, literally, means horny goat weed. When we looked into hard wine to see if there could really be anything to it, we were surprised to find that there really was a long tradition of this herb's use for sexual difficulties. In traditional Chinese medicine, horny goat weed is used especially for improving sexual function, including impotence and fertility. It is held to "warm the kidneys," raising sexual energy in both men and women. Low kidney energy is often involved in sexual problems in Chinese medicine.

And we did find one suggestive study in which people with kidney failure who were on dialysis had their sex drives improve when they were given horny goat weed, compared to people who didn't get the herb[2]. There are also studies showing that horny goat weed can restore low levels of testosterone[3]. Helping impotence and raising testosterone without affecting estrogen, combined with an ability to lower blood pressure, may make horny goat weed an ideal herb for treating male impotence and promoting sperm production.

Horny goat weed's other name, barrenwood, may also be a clue to its powers.

So is there anything to hard wine? Bois bandé, eleuthero and horny goat weed . . . who knows? Hollis's partner might be right!

Gifiti

Another time, we were in Honduras and were told by the locals about a herbal remedy called gifiti that was used to improve desire and erections. It was a combination of woody-looking stuff. Sold in clear bottles, it looked like herbs and barks and nuts soaking in alcohol. One sip was supposed to make you rather virile. So we bought it and each took the one sip. There must be something wrong with us: we fell asleep. Certainly, it did relax us; we were tired and had a great sleep that night.

Bust Your Britches

James Duke tells of two herbal aphrodisiacs soaked in wine or rum that he found in his travels in Latin America[4]. One is called siete raices and the other rompe calzon. Rompe calzon rivals hard wine and horny goat weed as the best name for an aphrodisiac. It translates as "bust your britches," because of its reputation for producing big enough erections to . . . bust your britches! There are no studies here, only anecdotal claims. But it is interesting that the two formulae contain a common herb: clavohuasca (*Tynnanthus panurensis*). This herb hails from Peru.

Ashwagandha is a herb used for increasing the body's overall ability to deal with stress. It promotes well-being and enhances stamina. It helps to restore sexual chi, or energy. It is used for reduced levels of energy, including sexual energy, nervous tension, stress, and anxiety. So it is especially useful for sexual problems that are related to nervous tension. Ashwagandha is an Ayurvedic herb, the traditional medical practice of India, where it is used as an aphrodisiac. In India it is used for a rejuvenating drink. Modern science has found that it contains hormone precursors that can convert into human hormones and balance them as necessary[5].

Chastetree berry is not considered an aphrodisiac, but because it can balance hormones in both men and women, it can be used if sexual problems arise from out-of-balance hormones. This can occur especially in PMS, in midlife, with depression and anxiety, or with low-progesterone or high-estrogen problems. It does not stimulate libido. But, contrary to legend, it does not suppress it either. Roman women, it is said, would use chastetree berry to control their sexual desire as they waited out the long nights while their husbands were away at war. Medieval monks would use this herb, known then as monk's pepper, to keep their earthly desires in check. Today's name, chastetree berry, also belies this belief. But it is not true. So go ahead and use this great herb without fear if you need it.

Chocolate. Try telling most women that there isn't something erotic about chocolate. Men, too. Why? Because good chocolate contains a substance that acts on centres of the brain almost like sex, in a relaxing, antidepressant kind of way. Many women will take chocolate over sex. And the smart ones take both. Chocolate is also a source of antioxidants if you are using the good, pure dark chocolate. I was never a chocolate freak the way Ted is until we tasted the chocolate in Guatemala. Beautiful chocolate with a hint of ginger or chili, it was easily the best chocolate we have ever had. Wow! I finally understood what all the hype was about. According to herbalist Diana De Luca, chocolate was considered the most powerful sexual tonic and stimulant of all by the Aztecs of Mexico, who blended it with different combinations of chili, cinnamon, cloves, anise, and vanilla, not unlike the heavenly chocolate we had next door in Guatemala. De Luca says that Montezuma would drink goblets of a chocolate potion containing cayenne, cinnamon, and vanilla before going into his harem[6]. Anyway, how can you go wrong? It's chocolate!

CHOCOLATE WAS CONSIDERED THE MOST POWERFUL SEXUAL TONIC AND STIMULANT OF ALL BY THE AZTECS OF MEXICO, WHO BLENDED IT WITH DIFFERENT COMBINATIONS OF CHILI, CINNAMON, CLOVES, ANISE, AND VANILLA.

From chocolate to truffles, but of the mushroom variety this time. We found references to the Greeks and Romans esteeming this exotic mushroom as an aphrodisiac, but the real champion of this magic mushroom is the early nineteenth-century French politician, writer, epicure, and student of food Jean Anthelme Brillat-Savarin. In his work *The Physiology of Taste*, Brillat-Savarin attributed the value of the truffle to its effect on the "genesiac" sense. Brillat-Savarin described this sense as the sixth sense of physical love, which attracts the sexes to each other with the goal of reproduction. "The truffle was supposed to excite the genesiac sense," he says. "This I am sure is the chief quality of its perfection, and the predilection and preference evinced for it, so powerful is our servitude to this tyrannical and capricious sense . . . . The truffle is a positive aphrodisiac and, under certain circumstances, makes women kinder, and men more amiable." He would go on to say, "Truffle. As soon as the word is spoken, it awakens lustful and erotic memories among the skirt-wearing sex and erotic and lustful memories among the beard-wearing sex . . . . it is still believed to bring about potency, the exercise of which brings sexual pleasure."

And now from Europe back to Latin America, where damiana* is considered an aphrodisiac used for lowered libido in men or women. This herb has a reputation as a herb of passion that goes back to ancient times, especially among the people of Mexico. It is native to South and Central America, and perhaps this is how it originally got its reputation for being a hot-blooded herb. Its original botanical name was *Turnera aphrodisiaca*—a dead giveaway for what this herb was believed to do! The Aztecs considered this aphrodisiac herb to be second in potency only to chocolate[7]. It is known to strengthen the reproductive systems of both men and women and to help restore diminished sexual vitality. It is a herb that calms and nourishes the nervous system, making it good for treating nervous conditions, such as burn-out, depression, and anxiety, that are related to sexual problems. It is used for impotence and infertility. In Mexico, it is made into a popular liqueur and sold in suggestive bottles that reveal what it is for. One of our favourite herbalists, Rosemary Gladstar, tells a story of how she made herbal balls containing damiana for a cruise ship of older people. They were so popular that they went quickly, and there were a lot of happy people on board, no doubt. Later, after the cruise was over, she was recognized as the lady who made these incredible herbal balls and was asked to make more of them for people that she ran into. Diana De Luca says that in parts of Mexico, a damiana cordial is still given as a gift by hopeful mothers-in-law who are impatient to be grandmothers.

Several foods have been considered aphrodisiacs. Though less exotic and sensual than chocolate or truffles, several varieties of beans top the charts. Cicero is said to have had his passion flamed by the common fava bean*, a legume with an ancient reputation as an aphrodisiac. And, as you will see in the section on male impotence, though the bean's legendary power may be somewhat enlarged, it just might do some enlarging for you also. Another bean with the same useful component as the fava bean is the velvet bean. Duke says that in Panama, the seeds of the velvet bean are believed to be an aphrodisiac.

Chocolate we get; truffles are exotic; we'll even accept the bean. But onions?! Yup, the onion has a long tradition as perhaps the unlikeliest aphrodisiac of them all. Today the onion has made toothpaste one of the most powerful aphrodisiacs, but, once upon a time, it seems that the onion incited kisses.

Fenugreek is considered an aphrodisiac and rejuvenator. Traditional Chinese herbalists used fenugreek for conditions of the male reproductive tract, and a famous nineteenth-century female reproductive tonic by Lydia Pinkham contained fenugreek seeds. Fenugreek has mild estrogenic effects. Once fed to harem women to enlarge their breasts, fenugreek seed and sprouts may actually do this, according to James Duke. You can take it as a tea, he says, or massage fenugreek powder on the breasts.

Two other culinary herbs with estrogenic effects and traditional reputations for enhancing libido are fennel and parsley.

Fo ti (ho shou wu), is a Chinese wonder herb known to increase vitality and sexual activity well into old age. Chinese herbalists have used fo ti to increase sperm count since ancient times. It strengthens the kidneys, blood, and liver and is reputed to give men the ability to produce children well into their eighties. Chinese legend tells of an elderly man unable to father children who, upon taking fo ti, went on to live 160 years and father 130 children. It is a rejuvenating tonic that will restore energy, increase fertility, and maintain strength. It even turns prematurely gray hair back to its original colour. It strengthens the muscles, tendons, ligaments, and bones. Linda has seen this herb do wonders to stop premature aging.

CHINESE LEGEND TELLS OF AN ELDERLY MAN UNABLE TO FATHER CHILDREN WHO, UPON TAKING FO TI, WENT ON TO LIVE 160 YEARS AND FATHER 130 CHILDREN.

Another Chinese herb with a reputation for increasing sperm production and fighting aging is goji berry*.

Ginger is reputed to be an aphrodisiac and is used for stagnation/congestion in the pelvic/reproductive region and to increase circulation to the pelvic region and reproductive organs. It is used for both men and women. Duke says he saw women in the markets of Peru selling "'hot' ginger to warm up 'cold' women"[8]. It is also used topically to warm cold kidneys.

Cardamom contains androgenic (male sex hormone) compounds and compounds that stimulate the nervous system, according to Duke. Arabic cultures have prized cardamom as an aphrodisiac for centuries. They often mix it into coffee, which is also considered in Arab countries to be a sex stimulant. Several other caffeine sources are also considered aphrodisiacs, probably because of their stimulant properties. In Brazil, guarana is considered an aphrodisiac. Jamaicans and West Africans consider the caffeine-bearing herb, cola, an aphrodisiac. And, of course, chocolate also contains caffeine. Just be careful of the negative effects of caffeine on your health.

Ginseng* also belongs on this list, as it can help to increase sex drive and libido. It is used for sexual inadequacy, especially when due to exhaustion and stress. It builds sexual vitality. Eleuthero (formerly Siberian ginseng) has a long history of use in stimulation of male virility. It is often used as a tonic for male reproductive systems. It increases stamina and rebuilds energy lost to exhaustion and adrenal depletion. Though more reputed as an aphrodisiac for men, there are reports of its sexual enhancement in women, too.

Sometimes called the female ginseng—though it's not—dong quai is considered by traditional Chinese medicine to be an all-purpose sexual and reproductive tonic for women.

Licorice is used for the reproductive systems of both men and women. It can aid in balancing hormones, so it can be used for reproductive issues. It is very good for adrenal exhaustion and for midlife crisis in men as well. It is also great for menopause and low progesterone.

Another licorice-tasting herb, anise is held by traditional folklore to increase libido in women and in men. The latter claim is far odder than the former, since anise is an estrogenic herb.

Oats is used to treat low sexual vitality, depression, and anxiety. It works for stallions! And there is some research suggesting it may work for human stallions, too. The reputation of oats as an aphrodisiac is long and well-established, hence the saying, "sow your wild oats."

Another herb that has traditionally been used when depression and anxiety are involved is the relaxing herb vervain. Duke says that this herb was used to treat any female reproductive problem associated with depression or anxiety.

Muira puama* is a mild aphrodisiac especially for women, but it is also used for impotence in men. This herb comes from Brazil, but it is so popular as an aphrodisiac that it has spread throughout South America and the world. It is a much-used remedy for men who are unable to attain or maintain an erection. It is used for impotence and depressed sexual activity. It is often referred to as potency wood. Not hard to figure out what this one means. It is also a nervine.

Another South American aphrodisiac is maca*. This herb hails from the high altitudes of the Peruvian Andes where it has been used by the Inca and others for at least two thousand years and perhaps much more. This cruciferous vegetable was cooked and eaten by both men and women to increase fertility, sexuality, and energy.

Nettle is used to strengthen the reproductive system and for weak kidneys. Herbalist Juliette de Baïracli Levy says that it cures infertility. She also says that mint was esteemed as a cure for frigidity, or lack of sexual desire, in both sexes and that it is still used today in Arab culture to ensure virility. Other culinary herbs that Levy lists include sage, which she says restores virility; watercress, which she says cures infertility; and summer savory, which, according to Levy, was much used as a tonic for people who are frigid and lack virility.

Pumpkin seeds are used to improve prostate heath. The seeds are loaded with zinc*.

Pygeum* is used to treat enlarged prostate, infertility, impotence, and sterility due to insufficient prostate secretions. In Cameroon, this herb has a long history of being used by traditional healers for "men's problems." They also used it for infertility as well as for menstrual disorders and as a general health tonic[9].

Rhodiola* can improve endurance and enhance libido. It has a long history of use by northern peoples to enhance fertility and treat impotence.

Red raspberry leaf is used to strengthen the genito-urinary system. It is a great nourishing reproductive tonic for both women and men.

Sarsaparilla is used for hormonal imbalances. There is a tradition of using sarsaparilla as a sexual energy enhancer for men.

Sassafras is used to balance male hormones.

Saw palmetto* is best known for its ability to treat enlarged prostate (BPH), cystitis, and bladder problems. But in the 1800s, it was considered an aphrodisiac and was used for impotence in men and for rekindling libido in both sexes.

Yohimbe is a traditional African aphrodisiac. It is traditionally considered one of the strongest aphrodisiacs for both men and women. It was used in tribal marriage rituals in Africa. Yohimbine, a component of this herb, is one of the only recognized pharmaceutical products for impotence. It works by dilating the blood vessels of the skin and mucous membranes, causing the blood to rise closer to the surface of the sex organs. So it is used for impotence, frigidity, and for stimulating an erection. This herbal aphrodisiac works as an erection-booster, but because of its myriad side effects and difficulty in working with it, we generally do not recommend yohimbe; though powerful, this is a herb to avoid.

In Bulgaria, tribulus, or puncturevine, has a reputation for enhancing sex drive and sexual performance in men as well as for increasing sperm production and fertility[10]. It was used in the Ayurvedic tradition of India for impotence and for the involuntary discharge of semen without an orgasm. Modern preliminary studies may back these claims up as they have found the herb has benefit for impotence and for male and female infertility[11].

Wild yam is used for liver congestion and for hormonal imbalances.

The pomegranate, with all its seeds, symbolized life, fertility, and abundance among several peoples, including Jews, Christians, Muslims, and Chinese. However, among the ancient Greeks, it also symbolized death and the under-world. Both these connotations have been represented in folkloric medicine with pomegranate being used both as a fertility treatment and, perhaps even more prominently, as a contraceptive.

APHRODISIACS & APHRODITE

The word *aphrodisiac* is derived from the name of the Greek goddess Aphrodite, the goddess of love and beauty. She possessed a kind of aphrodisiac—a magical girdle that irresistibly enticed men.

According to one version of her story, told by Hesiod, when the god of the sky, Uranus, came to lie with his wife, the earth goddess Ge, their son, Cronus, conspiring with his mother against his evil father, in perhaps the first enactment of Freud's Oedipus complex, ambushed his father and cut off his genitals. Cronus cast the genitals into the swelling sea, where a white foam arose around them. From the foam created from the seed of the sky god's genitals, a maiden emerged, a beautiful goddess whom men called Aphrodite, the foam-born goddess (*aphros* in ancient Greek means *foam of the sea*).

ENDNOTES

1. Lewis, Walter H., Memory P.F. Elvin-Lewis. Medical Botany: Plants Affecting Human Health, 2nd ed. Hoboken, NJ: John Wiley & Sons, 2003, pp.536–39.

2. Liao, H.J., X.M. Chen, W.G. Li. "Effect of *Epimedium sagittatum* on quality of life and cellular immunity in patients of hemodialysis maintenance." *Zhongguo Zhong XiYi Jie He Za Zhi,* 1995; 15:202–204.

3. Low, W.Y. "Asian traditional medicine for erectile dysfunction." *J Men Health Gender,* 2007; 4:245–50.

4. Duke, James A. *The Green Pharmacy.* NewYork: St. Martin's, 1998, p. 230.

5. *Withania somnifera* Monograph. *Alt Med Rev,* 2004; 9(2):211–14.

6. De Luca, Diana. *Botanica Erotica.* Rochester, VT: Healing Arts Press, 1998, p. 29.

7. ————, *Botanica Erotica.* Rochester, VT: Healing Arts Press, 1998, p. 29.

8. Duke, James A. *The Green Pharmacy.* NewYork : St. Martin's, 1998, p. 352.

9. Stewart K. "The African cherry (*Prunus africana*): From hoe-handles to the international herb market." *Economic Botany*, 2003; 57(4):559–569.

10. Mindell, Earl. *Earl Mindell's Supplement Bible.* NewYork: Fireside, 1998, pp. 127–28.

11. Mills, Simon, Kerry Bone. *The Essential Guide to Herbal Safety*. St. Louis MS: Elsevier, 2005, p. 606.

Part II

The Big Three: Female Infertility, Erectile Dysfunction, and Male Infertility

Chapter Two

FEMALE INFERTILITY

When Julius Caesar first steps on the stage in William Shakespeare's play, his first words are commands regarding his wife's infertility:

> Calpurnia! . . .
> Calpurnia! . . .
> Stand you directly in Antony's way
> When he doth run his course. Antony. . .
> Forget not, in your speed, Antony
> To touch Calpurnia; for our elders say,
> The barren, touched in this holy chase,
> Shake off their sterile curse. (*Julius Caesar* 1.II.1-11).

The ritual Caesar describes is that of the Feast of Lupercal, a very ancient fertility rite. Priests would take strips of skin from a sacrificed goat, an animal reputed for its virility, and run around a course with it. Barren women would place themselves in position on the course to ensure that they would be struck by the strip, because anyone so struck miraculously had her fertility awakened.

Today, the way we treat female infertility has changed. The fact that it never occurred to Calpurnia's husband that he might be partially responsible has not! But more about that in the next chapter.

Having your body do what you want it to do with ease, and not with dis-ease, is always about having a healthy body that has everything in balance. This simple rule is true of moving without arthritis, thinking without Alzheimer's, our heart beating without cardiovascular disease, and getting energy from our food without diabetes. It is just as true for having a baby. And since balancing the body into a state of harmonious, flourishing health always starts with what we eat, it should come as no surprise—though it does, because we rarely think of it this way—that fertility is greatly affected by diet. If you're trying to have a baby, then, while you're getting your house ready, get your baby's first house ready, too—and the best way to do that is through diet.

Though it may be a surprise to find that there is a fertility diet as much as there is a diabetes diet or a cholesterol diet, the diet itself holds no surprises. And that's not surprising. Being fertile is an offspring of being healthy, so the diet that's good for your body is the diet that's good for fertility. As with virtually every specialty diet, we can honestly say that the fertility diet is the very same diet you—and everyone else—should be on anyway.

Eating for Two

So what's the diet? Starting in 1989, Dr. Walter Willett, Dr. Jorge Chavarro, and their colleagues at Harvard followed 18,555 women who were trying to become pregnant to see how what they ate affected their chances of becoming pregnant (the Nurses' Health Study). What they found was nothing short of . . . not surprising at all! When we got our first highly anticipated look at their research, Linda's first response was, "Yeah. That's exactly what I've been telling people in my clinic for years." What is ground-breakingly important about these researchers' work is not what they proved, but that they proved it. Up to now there has been an unbelievable scarcity of research on how what you eat affects fertility. So what natural healers have believed about food and fertility for generations has now been proven, and, once again, the role of science—as happens so often in herbalism and diet—is less to discover than to validate traditional knowledge.

TEN SIMPLE STEPS TOWARD FERTILITY

1. Avoid trans fatty acids
2. Increase unsaturated vegetable oils
3. Increase plant protein but decrease animal protein
4. Eat lots of whole grains and complex carbohydrates but not refined carbohydrates
5. Get lots of iron from plants, but avoid iron from meat
6. Drink lots of water, but stay away from sugary soda pop
7. If you drink milk, temporarily drink one glass of whole milk a day, not skim
8. Take a multivitamin that contains folic acid and other B vitamins
9. Aim for a healthy weight
10. Exercise

The Many Causes of Female Infertility

There is a dizzying variety of possible causes for female infertility. There may be an underlying condition that is causing difficulty in becoming pregnant— uterine fibroids, ovarian cysts, endometriosis, pelvic inflammatory disease (salpingitis), low thyroid, tilted uterus, or scar tissue. If your difficulty stems from one of these problems, the underlying condition will need to be addressed. Linda's book, *Smart Woman's Guide to PMS and Pain-free Periods* will help you to resolve these specific issues and so improve your fertility.

Your frustration could also be coming from hormonal imbalances, past use of the birth control pill, chemicals, radiation, being too under- or overweight. The cause could be an infection, stress, or simply being worn out. Eating disorders, nutritional deficiencies, and even allergies can lead to infertility. Or there may even be antibodies to sperm or fertilized eggs.

But for many women, the simple—or not so simple—cause of infertility is the inability to release a mature egg. This ovulatory infertility is responsible for about a third of all cases of infertility. Though the ten tips uncovered by the Nurses' Health Study may well help with the many conditions underlying infertility, they are especially powerful (or at least especially proven to be powerful) for the "uncaused cause" of infertility known as ovulatory infertility.

Fat and Fertility

Perhaps nothing in health promotion causes more confusion than the understanding of fats. Deceptively disguised under the single word *fat* is a whole constellation of entirely different things. Some are essential to life—your life and giving birth to a new life—and some are detrimental to both.

The story of what makes a fat a good fat or a bad fat is really the story of hydrogen. Fats contain long strings of carbon molecules. If every one of those carbon molecules is bound to as many hydrogen molecules as it can carry, then it is saturated with hydrogen. So that fat is a saturated fat. If one or more carbon molecules are not saturated with hydrogen, that fat is an unsaturated fat. If only one carbon molecule is unsaturated, the fat is a monounsaturated fat (from the Greek *mono*, meaning one); if more than one carbon molecule is unsaturated, the fat is a polyunsaturated fat (from the Greek *poly*, meaning many).

Saturated fats come primarily from animal foods like meat and dairy, and they are bad for you. Unsaturated fats, which come mostly from plant foods, are good.

The new buzzword in health—or, in this case, lack of health—is trans fatty acids. But trans fatty acids are nothing new. They are the hydrogenated or partially hydrogenated oils that have been lurking in your margarine, junk food, and packaged food for years. And now that you know the difference between healthy unsaturated fats and unhealthy saturated fats, you can easily see why hydrogenating a fat is bad for you. When food manufacturers take an unsaturated fat and add hydrogen to it, they hydrogenate it. In other words, they take a healthy unsaturated fat from vegetable oil and turn it into an unhealthy saturated fat.

Trans fats are unhealthy for a host of reasons. They interfere with your body's metabolism of the healthy essential fatty acids; they increase bad cholesterol, decrease good cholesterol, and increase your risk of heart disease. They also mess up your liver's ability to detoxify, and they increase your risk of cancer, diabetes, prostate disease, and obesity. They suppress immunity, contribute to low birth weight, poor quality and quantity of breast milk, and contribute to abnormal sperm. In children, trans fats seem to increase the risk of asthma, hay fever, and eczema.

So how much trans fat can you get away with eating? According to a 2002 report by the Institute of Medicine of the National Academy of Science, the answer is none: there is no known safe intake of trans fats. And it turns out that the answer is the same for your future baby.

The Nurses' Health Study found that trans fats are a powerful obstacle to fertility. The more you eat, the greater your chance of ovulatory infertility. Even eating just a small amount of trans fats in place of unsaturated fats or complex carbs seriously increases your chances of infertility[1]. Trans fats seem to do their dirty work in two ways. They increase inflammation, which interferes with ovulation and conception, and they increase your body's resistance to insulin, which increases blood sugar and insulin levels, which, in turn, reduces fertility. Saturated fats have these effects, too, so it is not surprising that the Nurses' Health Study found that saturated fats do not promote fertility.

INCREASING YOUR INTAKE OF TRANS FATS BY ONLY 2% AT THE EXPENSE OF MONOUNSATURATED FATS INCREASED YOUR RISK OF INFERTILITY BY A WHOPPING 131%!

Unsaturated fats, on the other hand, are anti-inflammatory and increase insulin sensitivity and blood-sugar control. So they have the opposite effect on fertility from trans fats: they improve your chances of getting pregnant.

Of all the dietary factors harmful for fertility, the researchers of the Nurses' Health Study found the worst was consumption of trans fats instead of monounsaturated fats. Increasing your intake of trans fats by only 2% at the expense of monounsaturated fats increased your risk of infertility by a whopping 131%!

And don't go back to your bad trans fat habit once you become pregnant; it now looks like trans fats increase your risk of miscarrying when you do get pregnant[2].

So cut out the trans fats, cut down the saturated fats, and go ahead and increase unsaturated fats such as olive oil, canola oil, and flaxseed oil.

Plant Protein and Animal Protein: The Powerful Protein Difference

Protein promotes infertility. Or at least that's the way it seems at first. Women who eat the most protein are 41% more likely to have ovulatory infertility than women who eat the least[3].

But when the researchers of the Nurses' Health Study took a more careful look at the data, they discovered something amazing. Not all proteins are alike. While women who ate the most animal protein were 39% more likely to suffer the frustration of ovulatory infertility than women who ate the least, women who ate the most plant protein were actually way less likely to be infertile than women who ate the least.

So, as with fats, you have to make the distinction between animal source and plant source: eating lots of animal-source protein hurts your chances of becoming pregnant, but eating lots of plant-source protein increases it. The study found that adding just one serving a day of red meat, chicken, or turkey increased the risk of ovulatory infertility by a third. On the flip side, replacing 25 grams of animal protein with 25 grams of plant protein reduced the risk of ovulatory infertility by an incredible 50%. This relatively small change is easy to make.

EATING LOTS OF ANIMAL-SOURCE PROTEIN HURTS YOUR CHANCES OF BECOMING PREGNANT, BUT EATING LOTS OF PLANT-SOURCE PROTEIN INCREASES IT.

By the way, this finding that it makes a difference whether your protein comes from plants or animals is not unique to fertility. Once again, what is good for future babies is good for current adults. Eating lots of animal protein contributes to osteoporosis, kidney disease, heart disease, and many cancers, but eating lots of plant protein doesn't; and a vegetarian diet protects you from all of them.

Carbohydrates: These Guys are Complex!

Next to the unfairly discriminated-against unsaturated fats typically being lumped together with the bad fats, nothing in health circles has been more maligned than the much misunderstood carbohydrate. And the blame lies largely with fad weight-loss diets that fail to distinguish between refined and complex carbohydrates. In their exuberance over the discovery of how bad refined carbs are for you, the creators of carb-killing high-protein diets killed *all* the carbs instead of only the bad ones.

There is no doubt that the quickly digested refined carbs are bad for your blood sugar, bad for your figure, and bad for you. But there is also no doubt that the fibre-rich and slowly digested complex carbs are crucial to every aspect of your health, from managing blood sugar to managing cholesterol to preventing constipation and cancer. And there is also no longer any doubt that refined carbs are bad for making babies and that fibre-rich complex carbs are fertility's friends.

Why is that so? What do carbs have to do with fertility? The same thing they have to do with diabetes and obesity. Carbs are crucial for determining blood-sugar and insulin levels. Sugar and refined carbs are bad for balancing blood sugar and fibre, and complex carbs are good for it. That's why eating whole grains rather than refined grains reduces your risk of diabetes[4]. A landmark study reported in the *New England Journal of Medicine* found that a high-fibre diet reduces glucose in a way similar to diabetes drugs[5]. And, as we saw with fats, high blood sugar and insulin impedes fertility.

Even if your blood-sugar levels are still within the normal range but at the high end, you are only half as likely to get pregnant as women with blood-sugar levels in the low end of the normal range[6]. The Nurses' Health Study found that women who ate the most refined and quickly digested carbs—as opposed to whole grains and other good carbs—were 92% more likely to suffer from ovulatory infertility than women who ate the least refined and quickly digested carbs[7].

So, as with fats and proteins, not all carbs are alike; a distinction has to be made. Quickly digested refined carbs and sugars increase your odds of not having a baby due to ovulatory infertility. But slowly digested fibre-rich carbs decrease your risk of ovulatory infertility and improve your chances of having a baby.

And, before we leave carbs completely, one more negative note on the re-fined variety. When the bran and the germ are stripped away in the process of refining a grain, not only is the crucial blood-sugar-balancing fibre stripped away, so too are most of the B vitamins and iron. And, as we are about to see, that, too, contributes to infertility.

Ironing Out Infertility and B is for Baby

Folic acid is a member of the B-vitamin family. It is very well known that women who are trying to become pregnant need to supplement folic acid in order to prevent neural-tube defects such as spina bifida. Well, here's another reason for mothers-to-be to supplement folic acid: the same folic acid and iron that are stripped out of grains during the refining process are crucial for fertility.

The Nurses' Health Study found that women who take multivitamins long-term are 40% less likely to have ovulatory infertility than women who don't [8]. And they found that the biggest contribution was made by folic acid and iron. Women who got 700 mcg or more a day of folic acid from food and supplements were 40% to 50% less likely to struggle with ovulatory infertility than women who got less than 300 mcg a day. And women who regularly supplemented with between 40 and 80 mg a day of iron were also 40% less likely to have trouble getting pregnant.

But here's the surprise. As with fat and protein, it makes a huge difference whether your iron comes from animal-source foods or plant-source foods. Women who get most of their iron from meat (heme iron) do not receive the fertility benefits of iron that were found in the study. In fact, they may be at increased risk for infertility. Only women who get most of their iron from plant foods (nonheme iron) or from nonheme iron supplements receive the fertility-boosting effects of iron[9].

RICH SOURCES OF FOLIC ACID
LEAFY GREENS (SPINACH, KALE)
BEANS
BROCCOLI
ASPARAGUS
NUTS
WHOLE GRAINS

As an added bonus, one study has also found that taking vitamins containing folic acid and iron reduces your chances of having a miscarriage by 50% when you do become pregnant.

So, if you're having trouble becoming pregnant, check and see if your multivitamin/mineral contains at least 400 mcg of folic acid and 40 mg of iron.

Rich food sources of folic acid include leafy greens like spinach and kale, beans, broccoli, asparagus, nuts, and whole grains.

Beverages and Babies
If what you eat affects fertility, does what you drink affect it, too? The answer is yes, but here the picture is less clear. The usual suspects, as with almost everything else, are caffeine and alcohol.

There is no doubt that heavily drinking alcohol is bad for fertility: it can put a full stop to your period, confuse your hormones, and increase your chances of a miscarriage if you do become pregnant. The effects of moderate drinking are less certain. Studies that have looked at women who drink around a glass of alcohol a day are pretty evenly split: about half find that even this level of alcohol drinking impairs fertility and about half don't.

So, although it is clear that you can't drink much, you may be able to enjoy a little. But just a little. And if you want to be sure, skip it; it's definitely not going to help. Perhaps the reason that a small amount of alcohol seems not to be such a culprit is that stress is a huge factor in infertility, and one glass of red wine, now and then, may help to temporarily reduce feelings of stress, although in the long run it can contribute to stress by increasing cortisol, which reduces the levels of serotonin and melatonin as well as making serotonin receptors in the brain less sensitive to the serotonin there is. Serotonin and melatonin are both important relaxing and mood enhancing neurotransmitters.

The caffeine picture is even more confusing. Coffee and caffeine interfere with fertility, according to several studies[10]. But some studies have not found any increased risk at all. The Nurses' Health Study—which was able to look only at the effect of one to three cups of coffee a day—found no negative effect for coffee drinking.

Some studies have found that, although caffeinated drinks do not cause ovulatory infertility, they are linked to infertility from other causes, such as tubal problems or endometriosis[11]. The Nurses' Health Study found a 20% increase in all causes of fertility for women who drank a lot of caffeine, though not in ovulatory infertility. But the surprise was that the culprit turned out to be, not coffee, but caffeinated soft drinks.

So they looked at soft drinks and ovulatory infertility, and the surprises continued to come. Women who drank two or more soft drinks a day were 50% more likely to have ovulatory infertility than women who drank less than one soft drink a week. But it didn't matter if the soft drink was caffeinated or not. So soft drinks really do affect fertility, but caffeine may not. But caffeine can alter your hormones and may contribute to other problems that can cause infertility, such as fibroids, cysts, and endometriosis.

But perhaps all of this does not let caffeine off the hook. Several studies have found an association between drinking caffeinated drinks while pregnant and an increased risk of miscarriage[12]. A Canadian analysis of the research found that drinking only 150 mg a day of caffeine—that's about one to two cups of coffee—while pregnant increases the risk of miscarriage by 36%. It also found an increased risk of low birth weight[13].

So the bottom line is that you should definitely avoid soft drinks if you're trying to become pregnant, and you should probably avoid coffee it you want to play it safe.

Milk: The Fatter, the Better?

Have you ever wondered where your strong conviction that milk is good for you came from? The answer to that question lies not in the pages of this book, but in a book on highly successful marketing. But we can tell you where it didn't come from: a good book on science or health.

DID YOU KNOW?
MILK IS LINKED IN STUDIES TO TYPE I DIABETES, CELIAC DISEASE, ECZEMA, ULCERS, ASTHMA, AUTISM, BRONCHITIS, PMS, PAINFUL PERIODS, PARKINSON'S DISEASE, RHEUMATOID ARTHRITIS, ATHEROSCLEROSIS, BREAST CANCER, FATAL PROSTATE CANCER AND OVARIAN AND UTERINE CANCERS.

Milk is *not* nature's perfect food. Just ask any other mammal. No other animal drinks the milk of another species—milk is species-specific, produced by the mother as the perfect food for her baby—and no other animal drinks milk beyond infancy. The fatty fluid is fit only for the fast growth and weight gain of infancy.

Mother's milk is the perfect food for babies; cow's milk is disastrous for adults. Milk is a leading cause of allergies and ear infections. It is linked in studies to type I diabetes, celiac disease (watch for that one later in this chapter), eczema, ulcers, asthma, autism, bronchitis, PMS, painful periods, Parkinson's disease, rheumatoid arthritis, atherosclerosis, breast cancer, fatal prostate cancer, ovarian and uterine cancers, other cancers, and many more diseases. In addition to all these problems, the majority of people simply can't drink the stuff: about 75% of adults are lactose-intolerant.

And, despite the reputation and constant implications, high-quality, long-term studies consistently show that milk does not protect you from osteoporosis[14].

So nobody, including women who are trying to get pregnant, needs to drink milk. But if you are trying to get pregnant, and you do drink milk, then you should—get ready for this because it flies in the face of everything you have ever been told—drink one serving a day of whole fat milk—not skim, not two percent, but whole-fat[15]. This advice is not because the fat is good for fertility, because it's not, but because of the strange fact of what gets removed from milk along with the fat. Female sex hormones, like estrogen and progesterone, but only some male sex hormones are attracted to the fat globules in milk. So when you skim off the fat, you skim off these hormones, too, leaving behind some of the male sex hormones, prolactin, and insulin-like growth factor-1. These excess male hormones you are drinking get in the way of fertility. Prolactin, the hormone that stimulates breast milk, can suppress ovulation; that's why you usually don't get pregnant while you're breast-feeding (thank goodness!). Insulin-like growth factor-1 increases the ratio of testosterone to estrogen—not exactly a desirable blend for female fertility.

So, if you're going to drink milk, drink whole fat milk. And then, as soon as you get pregnant, stop; the stuff will kill you! Or consider drinking soy milk, a food that can help to balance hormones.

Weight: The Goldilocks Formula—This One's Too Fat; This One's Too Thin

Though we always hear about being overweight, when it comes to fertility, being underweight is just as bad. Being either overweight or underweight interferes with the normal menstrual cycle and throws off or completely stops ovulation. The Nurses' Health Study found that women with the highest and the lowest body mass indexes were more likely to struggle with ovulatory infertility than women in the middle[16]. The message is to hit your healthy weight.

If you don't eat enough, then, as your fat stores disappear, your menstruation and ovulation will first decline and then, eventually, stop altogether. Hence, the anorexic athlete who has no period (one study found that 16.7% of all infertile subjects had eating disorders). If you gain too much weight, you will experience a rise in insulin, insulin resistance, and insulin-like growth factor-1. These changes increase your testosterone and other "male" hormones (yes, women have some of these hormones, too). And, once again, increasing your male hormones is not exactly the way to go to increase female fertility.

The good news is that you don't have to go on life-changing diets; quite a small improvement in body weight can have quite a large impact on fertility.

Beyond Diet: Fertility Herbs and Vitamins
Chastetree Berry

The most important supplement to take for infertility is the excellent women's hormone-balancing herb chastetree berry. Although most chastetree berry studies have been on women's health issues other than infertility (it is the best answer in the world for PMS), several of them have also been struck by the power of that herb to help infertile women conceive[17]. In the most recent study, sixty-six women who had been unsuccessful in becoming pregnant for one to three years were given either a combination formula featuring chastetree berry or a placebo. Ten became pregnant while using the chastetree berry compared to half as many who were getting the placebo[18].

Chastetree berry may be especially effective when the infertility is related to a luteal-phase defect and elevated prolactin. Luteal-phase defect can cause infertility because a lack of the hormone progesterone prevents the uterine lining from developing properly. Two uncontrolled studies have confirmed chastetree berry's fertility power over luteal-phase defect. Combined, they looked at forty-five infertile women who had low progesterone levels. By the end of the three-month study, the herb had been successful in thirty-nine of the women. Twenty-five of them had normal progesterone levels, seven more tended toward normal, and—here is the big news—seven of them became pregnant[19].

In addition to chastetree berry, vitamin C can help women with this condition become pregnant; 750 mg of vitamin C a day helped 25% of women with luteal-phase defect become pregnant compared to only 11% of women who did not take vitamin C[20].

More Herbal Help

Though chastetree berry is the most important single herb for infertility, there are several other herbs, often taken in combinations that include chastetree berry, which can gently ease a woman's body back to fertility.

When the origins of infertility are hormonal, as they most often are, dong quai, red clover, licorice, wild yam, and squawvine are helpful along with the chastetree berry. Herbalist Kathi Keville says that several studies done in

China have shown that dong quai helps the ovaries function better and helps re-establish a normal cycle and fertility. If you are using dong quai, don't use it while you are menstruating.

Herbs such as valerian are often used for relaxing. Herbalist Amanda McQuade Crawford says that the calming herb skullcap is a reproductive relaxant that is really good for enhancing fertility. In Linda's clinic, relaxing herbs are almost always given for fertility because stress plays such a huge role—some say one of the biggest. We all know that when a woman has been trying for a long time to get pregnant, she feels a great deal of pressure. Many, unfortunately, even feel like failures if they cannot conceive. It is often the case that when a woman stops trying and decides to adopt, and the pressure is suddenly off, then, like magic, she conceives.

Herbs that support the liver and help to detoxify and to get rid of excess estrogen in the body that can interfere with fertility are a good idea. Dandelion root, burdock root, and Oregon grape root are among those used, as are herbs that increase circulation to the pelvic area, such as prickly ash, ginger, and dong quai. Linda particularly likes to use false unicorn for weak uteruses that are having trouble holding the fertilized egg. Even immunity herbs such as astragalus are used to improve immune function, which can be important in infertility. Yarrow is a great fertility herb when infection is part of the problem, since it is an antimicrobial herb with a special affinity to the reproductive tract.

Ho shou wu is a herb that strengthens the whole system and is used to increase fertility even in older men and women. Red raspberry and alfalfa are also very good nourishing tonics. And, of course, ginseng, the king of herbs, is excellent for increasing vigour and sexual energy, and, when taken regularly, is a great help for infertility.

Traditional herbalists usually use combinations of herbs instead of single herbs so that the different actions of the herbs can act synergistically. One of our favourite herbalists, Rosemary Gladstar, recommends the following two formulae for female infertility:

Fertility Tonic
- 4 parts rehmannia
- 1 part astragalus
- 1 part dong quai
- 2 parts false unicorn root
- 3 parts wild yam
- 1 part chastetree berry

This formula is taken as a capsule or tincture three times a day. If you've never heard of rehmannia before, you're not alone. But this little-known herb is also referred to by another one of our favourite herbalists, Michael Tierra, as an important herb used for female infertility in Chinese herbalism. False unicorn root, another strange-sounding herb in this formula, has a long tradition of use for the female reproductive system, including being used by early North American medical healers for infertility.

Female Fertility Tea
- 3 parts wild yam
- 2 parts licorice
- 4 parts sassafras bark or root
- 1 part chastetree berry
- ½ part dong quai
- 1 part ginger
- 1 part cinnamon
- ½ part false unicorn root
- ¼ part orange peel
- pinch of stevia

This formula should be taken as a tea three to four times a day.

Keville suggests one teaspoon each of chastetree berry, dong quai, eleuthero (formerly known as Siberian ginseng), motherwort, crampbark, and wild yam.

Vitamins and minerals also have a role to play in restoring fertility. Nutritional deficiencies can be a cause of infertility, and double-blind research has shown that taking a multivitamin/mineral increases female fertility. Giving 200 IU of vitamin E to the woman and 100 IU to the man significantly increases fertility in infertile couples[21]. Certainly higher levels—like 400 IU—can also be taken. Though the hint has never been picked up by modern research, one very early study found that 100 mg of PABA—a distant relative of the B-vitamins—taken four times a day helped twelve out of sixteen infertile women to become pregnant[22]. And when women suffering from infertility and endometriosis were given either a placebo or 500 mg of propolis twice a day, pregnancies went up from 20% in the placebo group to 60% in the propolis group[23]. Traditional herbalists would also use herbs to clear out infections and stagnations for endometriosis and other scarring diseases of the gynecological tract. Herbs such as prickly ash, turmeric, astragalus, dandelion root, wild yam, pau d'arco, chastetree berry, shiitake mushrooms, and dong quai may be used, as well as flaxseed oil and B-vitamins. Sugar, caffeine, alcohol, refined foods, and foods such as wheat may need to be avoided.

For fertility, zinc can be key. Other useful nutrients include vitamin C, bioflavonoids, flaxseed oil, beta-carotene, magnesium, selenium, B6 folic acid, and B12.

Antioxidants can help to keep a woman's reproductive system healthy in many ways. Low levels of antioxidants mean high levels of free-radical damage and scar tissue that can interfere with conception. Antioxidants also improve immune function and help build healthy eggs.

The complex of B vitamins helps to normalize hormones and to detoxify the body of excess estrogen. Iron is also important because low levels of this mineral are associated with difficulty in getting pregnant[24]. Kelp adds valuable nutrients to your diet that can improve the reproductive system and, because it is loaded with iodine, it is great for supporting your thyroid, a vital gland for helping you become pregnant.

Probiotics, like acidophilus and bifidus, can also help when the infertility is related to endometriosis or candida. For candida, you may also have to follow a special diet and use supplements like grapefruit-seed extract to wipe out the bad yeast (see chapter on yeast infection; for information on endometriosis and other underlying female conditions, see Linda's *PMS and Pain-free Periods*).

Ancient Help: Acupuncture

Acupuncture can help when the infertility is caused by problems of ovulation; it has been shown to improve ovulation in 83% of women who are not ovulating[25]. Ear acupuncture has actually been shown to work as well as hormone therapy. Fifteen out of forty-five women in one study became pregnant in both the acupuncture and the hormone group, but unwanted side effects only occurred in the hormone group[26]. In another study, acupuncture outperformed the fertility drug clomiphene with a pregnancy rate of 65% to one of only 45% for the drug. Acupuncture can help correct hormonal imbalances and increase poor egg growth as well as improve the fertilized egg's ability to attach firmly to the uterus. It can also remove blockages and rebalance the body and prepare it for fertilization.

Lifestyle Changes

Two lifestyle changes are also important: if you smoke, stop, and if you don't exercise, start.

Smoking can lessen your chances of becoming pregnant[27a], perhaps by as much as a factor of three. Women who smoke also take longer to become pregnant and are more likely to miscarry when they do. New research also shows that women who smoke throughout their pregnancies have smaller babies who are at 1.6 times greater risk of being obese by age four. Smoking during pregnancy seems to impair skeletal growth and produce babies who are more likely to grow up to be shorter and overweight or obese[27b]. The good news is that quitting smoking during the first trimester eliminates these health risks to your fetus.

TWO LIFESTYLE CHANGES ARE ALSO IMPORTANT: IF YOU SMOKE, STOP, AND IF YOU DON'T EXERCISE, START.

Exercise can help your fertility unless you are already too thin. If you're too thin, then exercise works against you by putting the brakes on luteinizing-hormone production. When luteinizing hormone goes on strike, eggs don't mature properly and the endometrium is unprepared to receive the fertilized egg.

For everyone else, exercise helps. That may seem obvious since we've already seen that healthy weight loss helps and exercise is part of losing weight. But the benefits of exercise go well beyond weight loss. A lifetime of sitting in front of the TV and the computer leads to excesses of blood sugar and insulin, and we've already seen with fats and carbs what that does to your chances of becoming pregnant. Vigorous activity, on the other hand, increases your chances. Women who exercise vigorously have a lower risk of infertility, with women who do at least five hours a week faring the best[28].

And don't forget timing. Though timing may not be everything, it is something. Women are usually fertile starting six days before ovulation begins, peaking on the day of ovulation, and ending on the day after. Your odds of getting pregnant improve the closer you are to ovulation.

The Harder You Try, the Harder It Gets

It's unfair, but the harder a time you have getting pregnant, the more stressed about it you become and the harder you try, and the more stressed you are and the harder you try, the harder a time you will have getting pregnant. Christiane Northrup, M.D., cites studies going back to the 1930s that show focusing excessively on the goal of having a baby can actually cause the release of eggs that matured prematurely and are not yet ready to be fertilized. Stress, as well as depression and anxiety, get in the way of your becoming pregnant. That's one of the reasons that relaxing herbs such as skullcap and valerian and calming nutrients such as calcium and magnesium can aid infertility. Relaxation therapy can also help. Researchers at the Harvard Medical School conducted a study of 184 women who were undergoing fertility treatment. While only 20% of the control group became pregnant, 55% of the group of women who went for relaxation therapy, cognitive therapy, and stress reduction did[29]. This study is not an isolated fluke. Several studies have found this relationship between relaxation therapy and fertility[30]. Acupuncture can also help to relax the body.

Polycystic Ovary Syndrome: The Most Fertile Cause of Infertility

The most common cause of ovulatory infertility is polycystic ovary syndrome (PCOS). Women with PCOS suffer from at least two of the following:

- Elevated levels of male hormones
- Infrequent periods or lack of periods and ovulation
- Enlarged ovaries with lots of small cysts

PCOS is mainly caused by insulin resistance and excessive amounts of male hormones. Insulin resistance leads to levels of blood sugar and insulin that are too high. And, as we have seen over and over again, too much blood sugar and insulin lead to infertility. In women with PCOS, elevated insulin elevates testosterone, which stops eggs from being released.

SUPPLEMENTS FOR FERTILITY
N-ACETYL-CYSTEIN
INOSITOL
CALCIUM & VITAMIN D

PCOS is most common in overweight women, and being overweight makes the condition worse, so the first step to restoring fertility in PCOS is to work toward a healthy weight. Losing weight significantly reduces the causes of PCOS: blood-sugar control problems and elevated male hormones[31]. Luckily, fertility seems to be very sensitive to the body's weight. Earlier, we saw that small improvements in weight could lead to large improvements in fertility. The same is true for PCOS-induced infertility. Even modest weight loss can improve insulin sensitivity enough to lower testosterone sufficiently to restore ovulation[32].

Several supplements can also help. N-acetyl-cystein (NAC) can improve insulin sensitivity in women with PCOS[33]. Inositol, a relative of the B-family of vitamins, can be beneficial; 100 mg given twice a day to women with PCOS and infrequent periods leads to significant weight loss and significantly more periods[34]. When thirteen women with PCOS were given 1,500 mg of calcium and 50,000 IU of vitamin D once or twice a week for six months, seven of them normalized their menstrual cycles and two of them became pregnant[35a]. An even more impressive study has highlighted the use of vitamin D. Forty-six women with PCOS were given 20,000 IU of vitamin D a week for six months. Fifty percent of the women who suffered from menstrual irregularities improved and a quarter of those hoping to become pregnant did become pregnant during the study[35b].

One of the most exciting studies is on a form of inositol called myo-inositol. We've already seen that inositol can restore periods. This new study found that, too. When myo-inositol and folic acid were given to women with PCOS for six months, 88% of them restored at least one menstrual cycle and a full 72% of them maintained normal ovulation. And here's the amazing part: 40% of them became pregnant! The researchers concluded that the combination of myo-inositol and folic acid restores ovulation and fertility in most women with PCOS[36a].

A promising study has now also shown that maitake mushroom can help. When seventy-two women with PCOS were given a special kind of maitake known as maitake SX-fraction, 76.9% of them ovulated. That's a good result, though it was not quite as good as the result produced by the drug clomiphene citrate. But the really interesting thing about this study is that clomiphene citrate is the go-to drug for fertility for women with PCOS, but, in this study, maitake worked better. None of the eight women who wanted to become pregnant in the clomiphene group did, but two out of three women in the maitake group who wanted to become pregnant did[36b], suggesting that maitake could be a good choice for infertility caused by PCOS.

Green tea might also help. While obese women on a placebo continued to gain weight, women taking green tea lost a little. Fewer women in the green tea group continued to experience a lack of periods, though the difference was not significant[37]. Green tea might help by increasing a hormone that binds some of the testosterone, reducing it and some of the problems it causes[38].

And don't forget to call your acupuncturist, because electro-acupuncture has also been shown to help. In a study of twenty-four women with PCOS, nineteen of whom had been unresponsive to drug treatment, nine of them had good results from the acupuncture[39].

And finally, although there have been no studies, the herb saw palmetto berry has been used clinically to treat PCOS because of its anti-male hormone effect.

CELIAC DISEASE: DOING WAY MORE THAN YOU MIGHT THINK

Celiac disease is an auto-immune response to the gluten in certain grains. Though better known as a disease that causes stomach and intestinal pain, celiac disease that is lurking undiagnosed may actually be the cause of as much as 8% of all unexplained infertility. In women, it can cause problems with ovulation, leading to difficulty getting pregnant; in men, it can cause low levels of the male hormone, testosterone, and high levels of the female hormone, FSH, and interfere with sperm production. So get tested for celiac disease. Simply avoiding gluten can sometimes jump-start fertility in both men and women.

Avoiding gluten means avoiding all forms of wheat—including kamut and spelt—as well as barley and rye. Rice and buckwheat are okay. Corn and millet do not cause celiac disease but may aggravate symptoms in sensitive people. Some sources feel that even rice and buckwheat can do this—so watch for symptoms.

Though most sources continue to list oats with wheat, rye, and barley, recent better-designed studies have shown that most celiacs actually do tolerate moderate amounts of oats just fine. Be careful, though: it is very common for commercial oats products to be contaminated with gluten. When people who thought they were on a gluten-free diet were put on a truly gluten-free diet, 77% of them improved!

If eliminating gluten doesn't resolve the celiac disease, then get tested for zinc deficiency. Celiacs don't respond to a gluten-free diet if there is a zinc deficiency, and zinc deficiencies are common among celiacs.

Drinking cow's milk early in a child's life is a major causative factor in celiac disease, and milk and all milk products should be eliminated along with gluten until the intestines return to normal.

Because celiac disease leads to malabsorption, celiacs often develop deficiencies of vitamins E, D, K, B12, and folic acid, iron, selenium, zinc, calcium, magnesium, carnitine, and essential fatty acids. So taking a high-potency multivitamin/mineral is a very good idea. Additional supplementation of particular deficiencies may also be necessary. As well as contributing to infertility, celiac disease in women who do become pregnant puts them at much higher risk of having babies with neural-tube defects, so taking folic acid during child-bearing years is very important.

There are a few other nutrients that can help celiacs. Glutamine helps to rebuild the damaged intestines and probiotics help to re-establish healthy microflora. Papain, the protein-digesting enzyme from papaya, seems to digest gluten and render it harmless to celiacs. So it may be a good insurance policy to take 500-1,000 mg with meals in case of hidden gluten. Whether these additional steps will help you get pregnant, we don't know, but they will help you feel better.

MAGICAL AND MYSTERIOUS MANDRAKE

The herb mandrake is soaked in mystery and lore. In early folklore, legend, and magic it is a love charm[40]. It probably makes its earliest appearance in the book of Genesis. Its biblical Hebrew name is *duda 'im*, meaning love plant or love-producing. R. K. Harrison of Western University says that the root of the word (no play on words intended) is *dwd*, meaning to love or to fondle[41]. In the very confusing, ambiguous, and magically suggestive passage in Genesis, Reuben finds mandrakes in the field and gives them to his mother, Leah. Her sister Rachel desires the mandrakes and asks Leah to give them to her (30:14). Leah protests that Rachel has already stolen her husband; does she have to steal her son's mandrakes, too? Rachel then proposes an exchange: you give me Reuben's mandrakes, and I'll give you Jacob for one night (that's some valuable herb!) (30:15). Leah agrees and says to Jacob, "Thou must come in unto me; for surely I have hired thee with my son's mandrakes" (30:16); "And he lay with her that night" (30:16). And the herb seems to act as a cure for barrenness because Leah, who has "left bearing" (29:35), conceives a child (30:17). The exchange of the magical mandrake so cloaked in confusion in this passage surely seems to have some aphrodisiac and fertility powers.

The mandrake makes a biblical appearance as an aphrodisiac a second time in the love songs of the Song of Solomon. When the poet invites her lover with the promise that "there I will give thee my loves" (7:12), her enticement includes the promise that at her gates, where she has put out all sorts of pleasant fruits, is the smell of the mandrake (7:13).

In ancient times, the fruit of the mandrake was eaten by barren women as a stimulant to sexual pleasure and the root was worn or carried as a talisman to ensure fertility. Some said to soak the seeds in white wine. Apparently, the magical fertility power of the mandrake remained in the lore of the medieval Jews, with references showing up in thirteenth- and fifteenth-century texts. We came across one claim that nineteenth-century Moroccan Jews put mandrake root over the fire and then bent over, allowing the smoke to enter their private parts and work its magic—a tricky position that you should be careful of trying at home.

The ancient Greeks, too, thought that mandrake possessed aphrodisiac powers. Harrison says that Dioscorides identified mandrake with the "plant of Circe" that was said to enchant you to sexual activity[42]. Circe, of course, was the witch who managed to seduce Odysseus to live with her for a year and who bore his child despite Odysseus's being in such a hurry to return to his wife and despite the fact that Circe had turned half of Odysseus's men into pigs. If the "plant of Circe" was mandrake, that's one powerfully bewitching aphrodisiac!

According to the Royal Society of Medicine, the belief in mandrake's fertility powers gained credence from the medieval doctrine of signatures[43]. This doctrine holds that God gave physical characteristics to plants as signs to reveal their healing values. The mandrake root looks like a man and so was held to have reproductive power. Apparently it was held that some mandrake roots were female and some male, depending on the anatomy of whichever gender they most resembled[44].

The medieval reputation of mandrake survives in the early sixteenth-century play of Machiavelli's named after that herb, *Mandragora* (*Mandragora officinarum* is the plant's botanical name). In Machiavelli's play, Callimaco says, "Then you must understand this: that there is nothing more certain to bring a woman to pregnancy than to give her a potion made from mandragora"[45].

It even makes an appearance in Harry Potter, although not for fertility, but as one powerful herb.

TREATMENT SUMMARY

Diet & Lifestyle

- Increase unsaturated fat; reduce saturated fat; eliminate trans fats
- Increase plant protein; decrease animal protein
- Increase fibre-rich complex carbs; eliminate refined carbs
- Get lots of iron from plants; avoid iron from animals
- Drink lots of water; eliminate sugary soft drinks
- If you drink milk, drink whole milk, not skim milk, once a day
- Reduce or eliminate alcohol
- Stop smoking
- Exercise
- Reduce the stress of trying too hard to have a baby
- Acupuncture

Nutritional Supplements

- Multivitamin
- Vitamin E: 200-400IU
- Zinc: 30-45mg
- Antioxidants
- If your infertility is related to luteal phase defect, add 750mg of vitamin C

Herbs

- Chastetree berry: 175-225mg extract standardized for 0.5% agnuside 1-2 times a day
- If the cause is hormonal, add one, or a combination of
  - Dong quai: 1-4g three times a day; 2-4ml tincture three times a day; or 1ml extract three times a day
  - Red clover: 2-4g or 2-4ml tincture three times a day
  - Licorice: 1-2g three times a day
  - Wild yam: 1g three times a day or 2-4ml tincture three times a day
  - Squaw vine: 1-2ml tincture three times a day
- Support the liver with dandelion root: 5-10ml tincture three times a day or 2-8g decocted as a tea three times a day
- For stress, add skullcap: 3g one to three times a day or 2-4ml tincture three times a day

ENDNOTES

1. Chavarro, J.E., J. W. Rich-Edwards, B. Rosner, W. C. Willett. Dietary fatty acid intakes and the risk of ovulatory infertility. *Am J Clin Nutr* 2007; 85:231–37.

2. Morrison, J.A., C. J. Glueck, P. Wang. Dietary trans fatty acid intake is associated with increased fetal loss. *Steril Fertil* 2008; 90:385–90.

3. Chavarro, J. E., J. W. Rich-Edwards, B. Rosner, W. C. Willett. Protein intake and ovulatory infertility. *American Journal of Obstetrics and Gynecology* 2007; in press.

4. Liu, S., *et al.* A prospective study of whole-grain intake and risk of type 2 diabetes mellitus in US women. *American Journal of Public Health* 2000; 90:1409–15.

5. Chandalia, M., *et al.* Beneficial effects of high dietary fiber intake in patients with type 2 diabetes mellitus. *New Engl J Med* 2000; 342:1392–98.

6. Hjolhund, N. H., *et al.* Is glycosylated haemoglobin a marker of fertility? A follow-up study of first-pregnancy planners. *Human Reproduction* 1999; 14:1478–82.

7. Chavarro, J. E., J. W. Rich-Edwards, B. Rosner, W. C. Willett. A prospective study of dietary carbohydrate quantity and quality in relation to risk of ovulatory infertility. *European Journal of Clinical Nutrition* 2007; in press.

8. Chavarro, J. E., J. W. Rich-Edwards, B. Rosner, W. C. Willett. Use of multivitamins, intake of B vitamins, and risk of ovulatory infertility: A prospective cohort study. *Fertility and Infertility*, 9 July, doi: 10.1016/j-fertn-stert.2007.03.089.

9. Iron intake and risk of ovulatory infertility. *Obstetrics and Gynecology* 2006; 108:1145–52.

10. Wilcox, A, C. Weinberg, D. Baird. Caffeinated beverages and decreased

fertility. *Lancet* 1988; 2:1453–56; Williams, M. A., *et al.* Coffee and delayed conception. *Lancet* 1990; 335:1603 [letter]; Hatch, E. E., M. B. Bracken. Association of delayed conception with caffeine consumption. *Am J Epidemiol* 1993; 138:1082–92; Grodstein, F., *et al.* Relation of female infertility to consumption of caffeinated beverages. *Am J Epidemiol* 1993; 137:1353–60; Stanton, C. K., R. H. Gray. Effects of caffeine consumption on delayed conception. *Am J Epidemiol* 1995; 142:1322–29.

11. Grodstein, F., *et al.* Relation of female infertility to consumption of caffeinated beverages. *Am J Epidemiol* 1993; 137:1353–60.

12. Srisuphan, W., M. B. Bracken. Caffeine consumption during pregnancy and association with late spontaneous abortion. *Am J Obstet Gynecol* 1986; Fenster, L., *et al.* Caffeine consumption during pregnancy and spontaneous abortion. *Epidemiology* 1991; 2:168–74; Infante-Rivard, C., *et al.* Fetal loss associated with caffeine intake before and during pregnancy. *JAMA* 1993; 270:2940–43; 154:14–20; Dlugosz, L., *et al.* Maternal caffeine consumption and spontaneous abortion: a prospective cohort study. *Epidemiology* 1996; 7:250–55; Weng, X., R. Odouli, D. Li. Maternal caffeine consumption during pregnancy and the risk of miscarriage: A prospective cohort study. *Am J Obstet Gynecol* 2008; 198:279.

13. Fernandes, O., *et al.* Moderate to heavy caffeine consumption during pregnancy and relationship to spontaneous abortion and abnormal fetal growth: a meta-analysis. *Reprod Toxicol* 1998; 12:435–44.

14. See, for example, Feskanich, D., *et al.* Milk, dietary calcium, and bone fractures in women: a 12-year prospective study. *Am J Public Health* 1997; 87:992–97.

15. Chavarro, J. E., J. W. Rich-Edwards, B. Rosner, W. C. Willett . A prospective study of dairy foods intake and anovulatory infertility. *Human Reproduction* 2007; 22:1340–47.

16. Rich-Edwards, J. W., D. Spiegelman, M. Garland, *et al.* Physical activity, body mass index, and ovulatory disorder infertility. *Epidemiology* 2002;

13:184–90; see also Green, B. B., N. S. Weiss, J. R. Daling. Risk of ovulatory infertility in relation to body weight. *Fertil Steril* 1988; 50:621–6.

17. Loch, E-G, H. Selle, N. Boblitz. Treatment of premenstrual syndrome with a phytopharmaceutical formulation containing *Vitex agnus castus*. *Journal of Women's Health & Gender-Based Medicine* 2000; 9:315–20; Propping, D., T. Katzorke. Treatment of corpus luteum insufficiency. *Z Allg Med* 1987; 63:932–33; *Gynakol* 1994; *Therapiewoche* 1993; *Therapeutikon* 1991.

18. Gerhard, I., *et al.* Mastodynon® for female infertility. Randomized, placebo-controlled, clinical double-blind study. *Forsch Komplementärmed* 1998; 5:272–78.

19. Propping, D., T. Katzorke. Treatment of corpus luteum insufficiency. *Z Allg Med* 1987; 63:932–3; Propping, D., T. Katzorke, L. Belkien. Diagnosis and therapy of corpus luteum deficiency in general practice. *Therepiewoche* 1988; 38:2992–3001.

20. Henmi, H., *et al.* Effects of ascorbic acid supplementation on serum progesterone levels in patients with a luteal phase defect. *Fertil Steril* 2003; 80:459–61.

21. Bayer, R. Treatment of infertility with vitamin E. *Int J Fertil* 1960; 5:70–78.

22. Sieve, B.F. The clinical effects of a new B-complex factor, para-aminobenzoic acid, on pigmentation and fertility. *South Med Surg* 1942; 104:135–39.

23. Ali, A. F. M., A. Awadallah. Bee propolis versus placebo in the treatment of infertility associated with minimal or mild endometriosis: a pilot randomized controlled trial. A modern trend. *Fertil Steril* 2003; 80(Suppl 3):S32.

24. Rushton, D. H., *et al.* Ferritin and fertility. *Lancet* 1991; 337:1554 [letter].

25. Mo, X., *et al.* Clinical studies on the mechanism for acupuncture stimula-

tion of ovulation. *J Tradit Chin Med* 1993; 13:115–19.

26. Gerhard, I., F. Postneek. Auricular acupuncture in the treatment of female infertility. *Gynecol Endocrinol* 1992; 6:171–81.

27a. Howe, G., *et al*. Effects of age, cigarette smoking, and other factors on fertility: findings in a large prospective study. *BMJ* 1985; 290:1697–99.

27b. Durmu B., *et al*. Parental smoking during pregnancy, early growth, and risk of obesity in preschool children: the Generation R Study. *Am J Clin Nutr* 2011;94:164–71.

28. Rich-Edwards, J. W., D. Spiegelman, M. Garland, *et al*. Physical activity, body mass index, and ovulatory disorder fertility. *Epidemiology* 2002; 13:184–90.

29. Domar, A., *et al*. The relationship between stress and infertility. *Fertil Steril* 2000; 74.

30. See, for example, Domar, A., *et al*. Impact of group psychological intervention on pregnancy rates in infertile women. *Fertil Steril* 2000; 73:805–11; Takashi, *et al*, 2002; Rodriguez *et al*, 1983.

31. Stamets, K., *et al*. A randomized trial of two types of short-term hypocaloric diets on weight loss in women with polycystic ovary syndrome. *Fertil Steril*. 2004; 81:630–637.

32. Ehrmann, D.A. Polycystic ovary syndrome. *N Engl J Med* 2005; 352:1223–26; see also Stamets, K., *et al*. A randomized trial of the effects of two types of short-term hypocaloric diets on weight loss in women with polycystic ovary syndrome. *Fertil Steril* 2004; 81:630–37.

33. Fulghesu, A. M., *et al*. N-acetyl-cystein treatment improves insulin sensitivity in women with polycystic ovary syndrome. *Fertil Steril* 2002; 77:1128–35.

34. Gerli, S., M. Mignosa, G. C. Di Renzo. Effects of inositol on ovarian function and metabolic factors in women with PCOS: a randomized double-blind placebo-controlled trial. *Eur Rev Med Pharmacol Sci* 2003; 7:151–59.

35a. Thys-Jacobs, S., *et al*. Vitamin D and calcium dysregulation in the polycystic ovarian syndrome. *Steroids* 1999; 430–35.

35b. Wehr, E, T. R. Pieber, B. Obermayer-Pietsch. Effect of vitamin D3 treatment on glucose metabolism and menstrual frequency in PCOS women—a pilot study. *J Endocrinol Invest* 2011 May 24 [Epub ahead of print].

36a. Papaleo, E., *et al*. Myo-inositol in patients with polycystic ovary syndrome: a novel method for ovulation induction. *Gynecol Endocrinol* 2007; 23:700–703.

36b. Chen J-T, *et al*. Maitake Mushroom (Grifola frondosa) Extract Induces Ovulation in Patients with Polycystic Ovary Syndrome: A Possible Monotherapy and a Combination Therapy After Failure with First-Line Clomiphene Citrate. *J Altern Complement Med* 2010; 16:1295–1299.

37. Chan, C. C., *et al*. Effects of Chinese green tea on weight and hormonal balance and biochemical profiles in obese patients with polycystic ovary syndrome—a randomized placebo-controlled trial. *J Soc Gynecol Investig* 2006; 13:63–68.

38. Hudson, T. Green tea and women's health. *Altern Complement Ther* 2007; 13:269–72.

39. Stener-Victorin, E., *et al*. Effects of electroacupuncture on ovulation in women with polycystic ovary syndrome. *Acta Obstet Gynecol Scand* 2000; 79:180–88.

40. Harrison, R. K. "The Mandrake and the Ancient World," *The Evangelical Quarterly* 1956; 28.2:89.

41. Harrison, R. K. "The Mandrake and the Ancient World," *The Evangelical*

Quarterly 1956; 28.2:91.

42. Harrison, R. K. "The Mandrake and the Ancient World," *The Evangelical Quarterly* 1956; 28.2:90.

43. Carter, A. J. Myths and mandrakes. *J R Soc Med* 2003; 96:144–47.

44. Bennet, B. C. "Doctrine of Signatures Through Two Millenia," *HerbalGram* #78, p.35.

45. Thanks to Ted's student Melanie Simon for pointing us to the use in Machiavelli.

Chapter Three

ERECTILE DYSFUNCTION (IMPOTENCE)

With all the media attention on erectile dysfunction lately, including the explosion of TV commercials for drugs that totally brighten your life by curing it, this very real problem would seem to be virtually epidemic. And it certainly is a growing problem! It is estimated that at least ten to twenty million men suffer from erectile dysfunction: the inability to attain or maintain an erection sufficient for

IT IS ESTIMATED THAT AT LEAST TEN TO TWENTY MILLION MEN SUFFER FROM ERECTILE DYSFUNCTION

satisfactory sexual function. And it is affecting men of all ages. Although 52% of men over the age of forty are at least partially affected, and 25% of men over the age of fifty suffer from it, it is not aging that directly causes this problem. Men are capable of retaining their sexual virility well into their eighties. In the very recent past, it was believed that virtually all causes of erectile dysfunction were psychological, that if you provided a stimulating partner, you provided a cure for the problem. But that was never true.

According to Terry Jones, of Monty Python fame, but also an historian, a medieval wife's complaint of her husband's failures in the marriage bed had to have such psychological causes ruled out. But how to do it? One twelfth-century manual suggests a physical examination of the husband's genitals by wise matrons. Jones says that witnesses would be summoned for a full-blown road test of the under-performing member. And lest you think the manual was joking, consider one Walter Defunt of Canterbury, whose wife, Jones reports, complained of his impotence. He was then "examined" by twelve worthy women who, upon completion of the exam, testified that his less-than-virile member was "useless." Another man, identified only as John, had his alleged impotence tested by having one woman expose her naked breasts and—according to court records, no less— hold John's member and embrace and frequently kiss him.

—*Terry Jones' Medieval Lives* (BBC 2004)

The Causes

We know now that the cause is usually physical and that there are many possible candidates: depression, stress, anxiety, fatigue, diabetes, hypothyroidism, prostate disorders, low testosterone or high estrogen, amongst others, can all be causes of impotence.

Cigarettes and Alcohol: Maybe This Will Make You Quit

Other causes include cigarette smoke and alcohol. If you smoke, you are more likely to experience erectile dysfunction than men who don't[1]. Put that on the cigarette box—that'll make men quit! Smoking just two cigarettes a day has been shown to inhibit erections produced by administration of a drug that dilates arteries and causes blood to flow to the penis[2]. Another study reported in Prescription for Nutritional Healing found that men who smoked a pack of cigarettes a day for five years were 15% more likely to suffer clogging of the arteries supplying the penis, leading to erectile dysfunction.

Alcohol, too, can cause erectile dysfunction since it can decrease testosterone production and cause your testicles to shrink. Seriously. Maybe that should go on the bottle, too! Though perhaps not as strong a cause as smoking, some of the same research that has indicted cigarettes has found alcohol to increase your odds of erectile dysfunction by 50%[3]. Strangely, the opposite has long been believed to be true: alcohol has an age-old reputation as an aphrodisiac that opens the way to sex. Although drinking a little may release sexual desire by breaking down inhibitions, the desire does little good without the ability, and, since drinking depresses the central nervous system, it also can take away the ability[4].

> Faith, sir, we were carousing till the second cock, and drink, sir, is a great provoker of three things . . . . [N]ose-painting, sleep, and urine. Lechery, sir, it provokes, and unprovokes: it provokes the desire, but it takes away the performance. Therefore much drink may be said to be an equivocator with lechery: it makes him, and it mars him; it sets him on, and it takes him off; it persuades him and disheartens him, makes him stand to and not stand to. In conclusion, equivocates him in a sleep, and giving him the lie, leaves him.
>
> —The Porter, *Macbeth* 2.III.22-32

Another factor that can be responsible for causing erectile dysfunction is prescription drugs; the most common drugs that cause this problem are blood-pressure-lowering drugs. Antidepressants and the ulcer medication cimetidine are also common pharmaceutical causes, as are the prostate drugs Finasteride and Flomax.

Atherosclerosis: The MI That Really Hurts (That's Male Impotence, Not Myocardial Infarction)

One of the major causes of erectile dysfunction in men is hardening of the artery walls that lead to the penis. It is well-known that when this same atherosclerosis causes a block in the blood flowing to the heart, you suffer a heart attack, and that when it causes a block to the brain, you suffer a stroke. Well, when it blocks blood flow to the penis, you experience erectile dysfunction.

And just like heart attacks and strokes, erectile dysfunction is on the rise in men. Atherosclerosis is the cause of erectile dysfunction in 50% of the men who suffer from it.

> "God gave men both a penis and a brain, but unfortunately not enough blood supply to run both at the same time."
>
> —Robin Williams

If you were told you had heart trouble, you would expect there to be some dietary changes needed to address the problem. Well, the same is true of erectile dysfunction. As Dean Ornish has shown, lifestyle changes alone can help to reverse atherosclerosis. In Ornish's study, people were placed on a vegetarian diet, used stress-reduction methods, and exercised. At the end of one year, there was significant reduction in atherosclerosis. Interestingly, the control group who followed the American Heart Association diet and regular medical care got worse. That's because a plant-based diet that is high in fibre, low in bad fats, and rich in good fats is the best protection against circulatory disease in the heart or the penis.

The Natural Approach
Drugs like Viagra tend to give instant results. So why use the herbal approach? Because the herbal approach goes deeper than the symptom, helping to correct your health by correcting the underlying problem. The natural approach improves the glandular system and the blood supply to erectile tissue and enhances nerve signals.

The natural approach is also safe. While Viagra works—sometimes too well—it is not without serious risks. Viagra frequently causes headaches and other minor side effects. But it can also cause abnormal hearing and vision. It can even cause loss of vision in one or both eyes that is sometimes temporary and sometimes—get this—permanent! Viagra also has serious drug interactions, especially with nitrates. But, most alarmingly, within two years of being introduced on the market, a study reported to the American College of Cardiologists found that there had already been 522 deaths from Viagra, most of them from cardiovascular events. What's really scary is that most of the men were under sixty-five and had no cardiac risk factors. In other words, healthy young men are having heart attacks and dying from using Viagra[5].

Nutrient Boosters

The overall energy and stamina required for sexual desire and performance requires an adequate supply of all the nutrients. But some, including the antioxidants and inositol hexaniacinate, are especially helpful supplements for erectile dysfunction. Antioxidants protect against atherosclerosis and, according to Michael Murray, N.D., inositol hexaniacinate not only reduces bad cholesterol, but also increases the blood flow to the penis, aiding in cases of erectile dysfunction. Other important cholesterol fighters that combat atherosclerosis and free up blood flow include red ginseng, sugar cane wax, guggulipids, red yeast extract, fibre, vitamins C and E, and L-carnitine.

The B-complex family of vitamins is especially important for energy, to help fight stress and to calm the nervous system. Several of the B vitamins are also crucial in preventing a build-up of homocystein, helping to prevent atherosclerosis and heart disease. Vitamin E is crucial to reproductive health, and zinc is vital to prostate health as well as being one of the most crucial nutrients for sexual function. Michael Murray, N.D., says that there is a lot of zinc in semen, so one way the body saves up zinc if there is a deficiency in the body is to gear down on sexual drive.

At least two studies show that the amino acid arginine may be promising[6]. For an erection to occur, the blood vessels to the penis need to dilate. That dilation depends on nitric oxide, and nitric oxide depends on arginine.

One placebo-controlled study found that Pycnogenol® helps[7]. Pycnogenol enhances the production of nitric oxide[8]. So what would happen if you put arginine and Pycnogenol together? Well, in one study, when 5% of men had developed the ability to achieve normal erections after being given arginine for a month, they then added Pycnogenol to the arginine for another two months. After the first month on the combination, 80% had normal erections, and after the second month, 92.5% did, making this a very promising combination[9a]. And now the promise has been confirmed by a more rigorously scientific double-blind study: 111 men with mild to moderate erectile dysfunction were given either a placebo or a combination of 40 mg of Pycnogenol and 1400 mg of arginine twice a day. After three months, the Pycnogenol and arginine group's score on the International Index of Erectile Function had gone up significantly from 15.2 to 25.2. The placebo group only improved from 15.1 to 19.1. And after six months, the Pycnogenol and arginine group's score had continued to rise to 27.1, while the placebo group had started to drop slightly to a score of 19. Compared to the placebo group, there was also a significant improvement in orgasmic function, sexual desire, intercourse satisfaction, and overall satisfaction in the Pycnogenol and arginine group. Testosterone levels increased from 15.9 to 18.9nmol/L, but barely at all in the placebo group[9b].

Herbal Help

Three of the best herbs for treating erectile dysfunction are Ginkgo biloba, muira puama, and ginseng. Ginkgo biloba is known for its ability to increase circulation to the extremities, including the head, hands, and feet. So why not the penis? For those who are suffering from erectile dysfunction caused by decreased blood flow, Ginkgo biloba can be just the thing. One study found that 50% of men who had not responded to conventional drug therapy regained potency after six months of Ginkgo biloba[10]. A second study has also proven ginkgo's effectiveness[11]. Research does show that ginkgo can resolve the difficulty by improving blood flow to the penis. Try taking 120 to 240 mg of standardized ginkgo. Results usually take at least twelve weeks.

THREE OF THE BEST HERBS FOR TREATING ERECTILE DYSFUNCTION ARE GINKGO BILOBA, MUIRA PUAMA, AND GINSENG.

But that is not all ginkgo can do. It can also help people on antidepressant drugs who suffer from loss of sexual desire or response, a common side effect of these drugs. In one study, 84% of men and women using ginkgo resolved the sexual dysfunction they were experiencing because of antidepressant drugs[12]. Since then, a second study was unable to reproduce this benefit[13].

A herb from Brazil that can be very helpful in treating erectile dysfunction is muira puama. Herbalist Michael Tierra mentions the root of this herb for impotency. Muira puama seems to be able to help with both the physical and psychological problems associated with impotency. A study done by Dr. Jacques Waynberg of the Institute of Sexology in Paris (yes, there really is such a place, and, yes, it really is in Paris) found that of 262 men suffering from erectile dysfunction or from lack of sexual desire, 62% of those with loss of desire were helped by muira puama and 51% of those with erectile dysfunction benefited from the herb[14]. Muira puama works because it is a nerve stimulant and aphrodisiac. Many traditional herbalists combine muira puama with other herbs that are designed to increase energy, glandular function, and sexual function. Herbs like ho shou wu, ginseng, damiana, astragalus, spirulina, saw palmetto, and raspberry are used. Clinically, Linda has seen these herbs work wonders when combined with lifestyle changes.

The herb generating the most excitement for erectile dysfunction now is Asian ginseng. Ginseng has traditionally been used as a treatment for impotence, but for a long time modern science has been sceptical. Not anymore. That all changed in 1995, when 1,800 mg of Korean red ginseng was discovered to improve erectile dysfunction significantly compared to both a placebo and a drug. The herb helped 60% of the men versus only 30% in the drug and placebo groups. Ginseng improved both the rigidity and the width of the erection, as well as improving libido as a bonus[15]. A year later, when thirty-five elderly men with erectile dysfunction were given either Korean red ginseng or a placebo, the herb once again defeated the placebo: ginseng helped a full 67% of the men, while only 28% of the placebo group improved[16]. In the most recent study, forty-five men with erectile dysfunction were given either 900 mg of powdered Korean red ginseng or a placebo three times a day for eight weeks. Sixty percent of the men on the ginseng had improved erections. Erection scores increased by 42% in the ginseng group compared to only 16% in the placebo group. Penile rigidity was significantly better in the ginseng group. Sexual function in the ginseng group improved by 36% versus 10.4% in the placebo group. And again, ginseng also improved their sexual desire[17].

In the first ever review of research on Korean red ginseng and erectile dysfunction, researchers found seven randomized, controlled studies that included 363 men. Six of those studies found that the ginseng improved erectile function more than the placebo did. Putting all the studies together into a meta-analysis, the researchers found that it was no placebo effect: the herb really works better than a placebo[18].

Another useful herb for male sexual vitality is eleuthero (formerly Siberian ginseng). Eleuthero is helpful for aiding in underdeveloped sex glands, impotence, and frigidity. Eleuthero has an ancient reputation for stimulating male virility. Rosemary Gladstar says it is commonly used as a male-reproductive-system tonic and recommends it when sexual energy is flagging due to exhaustion and adrenal depletion.

Though long used in Russia, Scandinavia, and Asia, *Rhodiola rosea* is having trouble getting the attention it deserves in North America. A wonderful herb for relaxing and calming you down while it simultaneously increases your mental and physical energy, Rhodiola just may have some sexual powers, too. When thirty-five men who suffered from erectile dysfunction, premature ejaculation, or both took 150 to 200 mg of Rhodiola for three months, twenty-six of them responded with substantially improved sexual function[19]. Rhodiola was used by the Vikings to enhance physical strength and endurance, and traditionally it has been used by many northern peoples to enhance fertility and treat impotence. And certainly the Vikings were no ordinary men.

RHODIOLA WAS USED BY THE VIKINGS TO ENHANCE PHYSICAL STRENGTH AND ENDURANCE, AND TRADITIONALLY IT HAS BEEN USED BY MANY NORTHERN PEOPLES TO ENHANCE FERTILITY AND TREAT IMPOTENCE.

Turning from northern herbs to southern herbs, you may remember damiana from the folklore, potions, and aphrodisiacs chapter. This herb has been esteemed as an aphrodisiac since ancient times, especially by Mexican cultures. Although there are not yet any clinical studies to test the ancient claims, the testimony of several leading modern herbalists suggests that this herb should be given a serious scientific look. Rosemary Gladstar and Diana De Luca both say that the herb really works. And Michael Tierra calls it a mild aphrodisiac for men and women. Michael Murray, N.D., explains that damiana is thought to slightly irritate the urethra, increasing the sensitivity of the penis. He says that a cup of damiana tea a day should do the trick.

Heading further south, we go from Mexico to Peru and to another herb you may recall from the folklore, potions, and aphrodisiacs chapter: maca. The first modern, scientific excitement over maca for erectile dysfunction came from promising research on psychological causes and on sexual dysfunction brought on by selective serotonin reuptake inhibitor (SSRI) antidepressants like Prozac.

When sixteen men and women who were suffering from major depression began to suffer from sexual dysfunction caused by their SSRIs, researchers tried giving them maca. On two scales of sexual function, maca produced significant improvement, and, according to one of the two scales, it also significantly improved libido. Maca significantly increased the frequency of what the researchers clinically called "sexual attempts and enjoyable experiences"[20]. So add maca to your list, along with ginkgo, of things to try if antidepressant drugs are keeping you down.

Maca can improve sexual desire in healthy men who are not on SSRIs, too. In a double-blind study of forty-five healthy men, maca improved their subjective evaluation of sexual desire[21]. And what better measure of sexual desire than subjective evaluation? At least one other study has found significant improvement in libido in healthy men[22a].

But the big news in maca research is that the herb has now been shown to help erectile dysfunction caused by physical problems as well as erectile dysfunction brought on as an adverse effect of antidepressant drugs. In a double-blind study, fifty young men with mild erectile dysfunction were given either 1,200 mg of pulverized and dehydrated maca root or a placebo twice a day for twelve weeks. Scores on the International Index of Erectile Function improved significantly more in the maca group than they did in the placebo group. Subjectively, scores on the Satisfaction Profile for psychological, physical, and social performance all improved significantly more on the maca than on the placebo[22b].

Though the case is not quite so clear for women, as you will see in the menopause section, in men, maca seems to do its work safely without affecting hormones[23a]. In this most recent study, maca once again delivered its benefits without significantly changing levels of follicle-stimulating hormone, luteinizing hormone, prolactin or testosterone.

Though long thought of as a mild aphrodisiac, a more unexpected herb on the male libido list is fenugreek. Male libido seems like a surprising use for a herb better known for its ability to affect the female hormone estrogen and for its ability to enlarge breasts. But you may remember from the folklore, potions, and aphrodisiacs chapter that traditional Chinese medicine also uses fenugreek for conditions of the male reproductive tract. And now a modern placebo-controlled study has confirmed that fenugreek effectively boosts male libido. Fifty-four men between the ages of twenty-five and fifty-two, who were suffering from low libido but no sexual dysfunction, were given either a placebo or 300 mg of fenugreek extract powder mixed with 17 mg of magnesium, 15 mg of zinc and 5 mg of B6. After six weeks, the fenugreek significantly improved in all four categories tested: sexual fantasy, sexual arousal, sexual behaviour/experience, and orgasm. The placebo group experienced no improvement at all; 81% of the men taking fenugreek said that their libido improved and 63% said the quality of their sexual performance improved. The placebo group reported no improvement in either of these categories[23b].

Other helpful herbs for increasing male sexual function are astragalus, sarsaparilla, saw palmetto, and yohimbe.

Acupuncture can also help to improve blood flow and overall health.

Strange and Not So Strange Lifestyle Tips
We've already seen that certain lifestyle changes, such as giving up smoking and drinking, can help. Well, here are some more strange, and not so strange, helpful lifestyle changes.

It should come as no surprise after reading the chapter on female fertility that diet plays a huge role in sexual and reproductive health. For men, too, sufficient levels of hormones and sufficient blood flow to the penis require a healthy diet. And a healthy diet means plenty of whole foods, including fruits, vegetables, whole grains, legumes, nuts, and seeds.

A couple of legumes in particular may be beneficial. The fava bean has an ancient reputation as an aphrodisiac. Cicero apparently believed that this bean was an inciter of passion. Well, there may just be something to it. Fava beans are a great source of L-dopa, and large amounts of the drug L-dopa are known to cause painful, long-lasting erections even when you are not sexually aroused. James Duke, Ph.D., says that, although fava beans can't do that (saving much embarrassment around the dinner table), a large serving may just pack

SNIFF TEST: SOME SMELLS THAT STIMULATE BLOOD FLOW TO THE PENIS

HOT CINNAMON BUNS
PUMPKIN PIE
LAVENDER
DOUGHNUTS
BLACK LICORICE
BUTTERED POPCORN

enough L-dopa to help you attain an erection. Only 250 mg of cooked fava beans has been shown to substantially increase blood levels of L-dopa[24].

Panamanians claim, according to Duke, that the seeds of the velvet bean are an aphrodisiac. And guess what? Velvet bean is loaded with L-dopa, too.

Not overdoing the protein is another way to boost L-dopa.

And here is perhaps the strangest erectile dysfunction study of all. Alan Hirsch, M.D., attached devices to men's penises to test their reactions to smells. That must have been the most surreal-looking laboratory of all. And who would have volunteered? Amazingly, Hirsch found that the smell of hot cinnamon buns caused the greatest spike in blood flow. Pumpkin pie, lavender, and, get this, doughnuts also boosted blood flow to the penis. When pumpkin pie and lavender were combined, penile blood flow went up by 40%! Black licorice was another biggie. And when it was combined into the classic combination of black licorice and doughnut, penile blood flow went up 31.5%. An oldie but a goody, the smell of pumpkin pie and doughnuts combined produced 20% boosts in blood flow. And how did Saturday night at the movies come to be the classic date? Maybe because the smell of buttered popcorn sent 9% more blood rushing to the penis! What will science discover next?

Coming back to the much more mundane—and there goes that buttered popcorn—trans fatty acids, those wreakers of havoc on female fertility, don't do the men any favours either. Trans fats disrupt blood-vessel linings, disturbing blood flow and contributing to erectile dysfunction. Essential fatty acids can help blood flow.

And finally, being overweight can lead to erectile dysfunction. A two-year study of obese men with erectile dysfunction found that a low-calorie diet combined with exercise significantly improved the problem. Thirty-one percent of them returned to normal[25]. Even independent of obesity, exercise can help. When sedentary but healthy men exercised, their libidos got a boost, as evidenced by an increased frequency of intimate activity, and their performance got a boost, as evidenced by increased reliability of sexual functioning and a higher percentage of satisfying orgasms[26]. Exercise can also increase blood count and flow, another reason it may help with erectile dysfunction. It also reduces anxiety and stress.

TREATMENT SUMMARY
Diet & Lifestyle
- Focus on fruit, vegetables, whole grains, legumes (especially fava beans), nuts, and seeds
- Eliminate trans fats and increase essential fatty acids
- Quit smoking
- Reduce alcohol
- Attain a healthy weight

Nutritional Supplements
- Inositol hexaniacinate: 1,000-3,000mg
- Pycnogenol: 40mg twice a day
- Arginine: 1,400mg twice a day
- Antioxidants

Herbs
Choose one or a combination of:
- Korean red ginseng: 900mg two to three times a day
- Ginkgo biloba: 240mg extract standardized for 6% terpene lactones and 24% ginkgoflavone glycosides
- Muira puama: 1-1.5g extract

- Maca: 1,200mg twice a day
- (If circulatory problems are involved, be sure to include Ginkgo; if stress is involved, be sure to include ginseng)
- Rhodiola rosea and damiana can also help

END NOTES

1. Condra, M., *et al*. Prevalence and significance of tobacco smoking in impotence. *Urology* 1986; 27:495–98; Marin-Morales, A., *et al*. Prevalence and independent risk factors for erectile dysfunction in Spain: Results of the *epidemiologia de la disfuncion erectile masculine* study. *J Urol* 166:569–75.

2. Morley, J. E. Management of impotence. *Postgrad Med* 1993; 93:65–72.

3. Marin-Morales, A., *et al*. Prevalence and independent risk factors for erectile dysfunction in Spain: Results of the *epidemiologia de la disfuncion erectile masculine* study. *J Urol* 166:569–75.

4. Lewis, Walter, Memory Elvin-Lewis, *Medical Botany: Plants Affecting Human Health*. Hoboken NJ: John Wiley & Sons 2003, p 535.

5. Kaul, S., *et al*. Report to the American College of Cardiologists, Anaheim CA, March 14, 2000.

6. Zorgniotti, A. W., E. F. Lizza. Effect of large doses of the nitric oxide precursor, L-arginine, on erectile dysfunction. *Int J Impot Res* 1994; 6:33–36; Chen, J., *et al*. Effect of oral administration of high-dose nitric oxide donor L-arginine in men with organic erectile dysfunction: results of a double-blind, randomized study. *BJU Int* 1999; 83:269–73.

7. Durackova, Z., *et al*. Lipid metabolism and erectile function improvement by Pycnogenol®, extract from the bark of *Pinus pinaster* in patients suffering from erectile dysfunction—a pilot study. *Nutr Res* 2003; 23:1189–98.

8. Fitzpatrick, D. F., *et al*. Endothelium-dependent vascular effects of Pycnogenol. *J Cardiovasc Pharmacol* 1998; 32:509-15; Hidaka T, *et al*. Pycnogenol®, French maritime pine bark extract, augments endothelium-dependent vasodilation in humans. *Hypertens Res*. Sep 2007; 30:775–780.

9a. Stanislavov, R., V. Nikolova. Treatment of erectile dysfunction with pycnogenol and L-arginine. *J Sex Marital Ther* 2003; 29:207–13.

9b. Ledda A, *et al*. Investigation of a complex plant extract for mild to moderate erectile dysfunction in a randomized, double-blind, placebo-controlled, parallel-arm study. *BJU Int* 2010; 106:1030–1033.

10. Sikora, R., *et al*. *Ginkgo biloba* extract in the therapy of erectile dysfunction. *J Urol* 1989; 141:188A.

11. Sohn, M., R. Sikora. Ginkgo biloba extract in the therapy of erectile dysfunction. *J Sec Educ Ther* 1991; 17:53–61.

12. Cohen, A.J., B. Bartlik. *Ginkgo biloba* for antidepressant-induced sexual dysfunction. *J Sex Marital Ther* 1998; 24:139–43.

13. Kang, B. J., *et al*. A placebo-controlled, double-blind trial of *Ginkgo biloba* for antidepressant-induced sexual dysfunction. *Hum Psychopharmacol* 2002; 17:279–84.

14. Waynberg, J. Contributions to the clinical validation of the traditional use of Ptychopetalum guyanna. Presented at the First International Congress on Ethnopharmacology, Strasbourg, France, June 5–9, 1990.

15. Choi, H. K., D. H. Seong, K. H. Rha. Clinical efficacy of Korean red ginseng for erectile dysfunction. *Int J Impot Res* 1995; 7:181–86.

16. *Korean J Ginseng Sci* 1996.

17. Hong, B., *et al*. A double-blind crossover study evaluating the efficacy of Korean red ginseng in patients with erectile dysfunction: A preliminary report. *The Journal of Urology* 2002; 168:2070–73.

18. Jang, D.-J., *et al*. Red ginseng for treating erectile dysfunction: a systematic review. *Br J Clin Pharmacol* 2008; 66:444–450.

19. Brown, R.P., et al. *Rhodiola rosea*: A phytomedicinal overview. *HerbalGram* #65.

20. Dording, C. M., *et al.* A double-blind, randomized, pilot dose-findings study of maca root (*L. meyenii*) for the management of SSRI-induced sexual dysfunction. *CNS Neurosci Ther* 2008; 14:182–91.

21. Gonzales, G. F., *et al.* Effect of *Lepidium meyenii* (Maca) on sexual desire and its absent relationships with serum testosterone levels in adult healthy men. *Andrologia* 2002; 34:367–72.

22a. Cordova, A., *et al.* Effecto del *Lepidium meyenii* (Maca) una planta alco-andina sobre el escado de animo y el deseo sexual en varones aparencemente normales. *Reproducao e Climaterio* 2001; 16:S96–S97.

22b. Zenico T, *et al.* Subjective effects of Lepidium meyenii (maca) extract on well-being and sexual performance in patients with mild erectile dysfunction: a randomized, double-blind clinical trial. *Andrologia* 2009; 41:95–99.

23a. Gonzales, G., *et al.* Effect of *Lepidium meyenii* (Maca), a root with aphrodisiac and fertility-enhancing properties, on serum reproductive hormone levels in adult healthy men. *Journal of Endocrinology* 2003; 176:163–68; Gonzales, G. F., *et al.* Effect of *Lepidium meyenii* (Maca) on sexual desire and its absent relationships with serum testosterone levels in adult healthy men. *Andrologia* 2002; 34:367–72.

23b. Steels E, A. Rao, L. Vitetta. Physiological aspects of male libido enhanced by standardized *Trigonella foenum-graecum* extract and mineral formulation. *Phytother Res* 2011 [epub ahead of print], doi:10.1002/ptr.3360.

24. Rabey, J. M., *et al.* Broad bean (*Vicia faba*) consumption and Parkinson's disease. *Adv Neurol* 1993; 60:681–84.

25. Esposito, K., *et al.* Effect of lifestyle changes on erectile dysfunction in obese men: a randomized control study. *JAMA* 2004; 291:2978–84.

26. White, J. R., *et al.* Enhanced sexual behavior in exercising men. *Arch Sex Behav* 1990; 19:193–209.

Chapter Four

MALE INFERTILITY

It's not easy being a sperm. You try to do one thing and do it well, and the odds of your reaching your goal are so small it's a wonder anyone gets there at all. There are a hundred to two hundred million sperm in the average ejaculation, and there may be as many as half a billion. And yet, the course they have to run is so hostile, so fraught with obstacles, that only about forty will ever get even close to the egg. So if conception is ever going to happen, there needs to be a lot of sperm trying, and they have to be very good at what they do. So the goal of maximizing fertility is increasing sperm count and, even more importantly, improving sperm quality. If your sperm cells are ever going to complete the course, they need to be very strong swimmers, and they need to be especially good at swimming rapidly in a straightforward linear direction; it's these guys that have the best chance of making it.

The testicles produce about a hundred million sperm cells a day. If there are over forty million of them per millilitre, that is considered normal, and your chances of conception are normal. If there are less than five million per millilitre, then fertility will become a struggle. Infertility is defined as the inability to conceive after one year of trying, though it can become frustrating long before that. As we have already seen, the male is the infertile partner about 40% of the time. In another 20% of cases, both partners contribute. When the male is the infertile one, it is usually because of low sperm count or quality. About 6% of all men between fifteen and fifty are infertile.

Why Are So Many Men Infertile?

There are many possible causes of infertility in men. The first may come as a surprise. Sperm are produced in the testes, and for production to work, the testes must be kept at a slightly lower temperature than the rest of the body. Sperm production requires that the temperature of the testes be carefully maintained at between 94°and 96° Fahrenheit. If the temperature peaks above 96°, sperm production slows down or even stops. The need to keep the testes cooler than the rest of the body is why they hang in the scrotum away from the body. Men who struggle with infertility usually have higher scrotal temperatures than fertile men. The good news is that now that you know this, simply reducing the temperature is often enough to end the infertility.

How do you lower the temperature of your testes? Frequent use of hot tubs and saunas and tight underwear and pants all cause the scrotum to be kept too warm. Infertile men should consider switching to boxers! Excessively vigorous exercise can also do it, with rowing machines, simulated cross-country skiing, treadmills, and jogging being the worst.

Obesity can also keep the testes too warm. Overweight men are less fertile than men who maintain a healthy weight. Carrying too much weight not only lowers sperm count by elevating the temperature of the testes, it also lowers testosterone and inhibits the production of sperm that are strong swimmers. A large study has found that as body mass index goes up in men, fertility goes down[1]. If obesity is the problem, see the chapter on weight loss.

Infections in a man's genito-urinary tract can also be the cause of infertility. If infection is the source of the problem, see the chapter on urinary tract infections.

Other possible causes include candida (see the chapter on candida), glandular diseases, heavy metals, and poor diets, too high in saturated fat and too low in fibre, that increase the estrogen in the body. Chemicals found in pesticides, plastics and other materials, and industrial chemicals have been found to mimic estrogen and to cause decreased sperm counts, infertility, undescended testes, and other developmental disorders of the male sexual system. Although a lot of attention has been paid to bisphenol A, or BPA, in certain plastics lately, the concern is actually not new. It has long been known that BPA, even in very small amounts, mimics estrogen in the body, and that, added to all the other external sources of estrogen, it could contribute to infertility and a whole host of hormonally sensitive conditions in men and women. And estrogen may be found not only in your water bottle, but in your water! Estrogen, perhaps from estrogen in birth control pills being secreted into the water system through urine, has actually been found in our drinking water[2]. All of these environmental factors have been steadily degrading the quality of sperm over the past several decades[3]. Sperm count and sperm quality have plummeted: sperm counts are only 40% of what they were in 1940[4]. That's scary; that's the stuff of science-fiction movies. What happens if that trend continues?

We have already seen the role celiac disease, an autoimmune reaction to the gluten in certain grains, can play in infertile women. Well, in men, it can cause low levels of the male hormone, testosterone, and high levels of the female hormone, FSH, and interfere with sperm production. Following a gluten-free diet has enabled some men to conceive when they previously could not.

Other causes of male infertility include smoking, alcohol, caffeine, recreational and pharmaceutical drugs, stress, and not getting enough exercise. Cigarette-smoking very clearly contributes both to low sperm counts and to sperm quality. Smoking leads to sperm with poorer motility (the sperm's ability to move on its own) and more frequent abnormalities[5]. Drinking too much alcohol also decreases the number of normal sperm[6] and gets in the way of sperm production. Drugs, both recreational and pharmaceutical, can also contribute to infertility. Marijuana, hash, and cocaine may lower sperm counts and cause

DID YOU KNOW?
MARIJUANA, HASH, AND COCAINE MAY CAUSE SPERM TO BE ABNORMALLY SHAPED.

sperm to be abnormally shaped. Pharmaceutical drugs can cause infertility in all kinds of creative ways. Sulfasalazine, cimetidine, and nitrofurantoin all interfere with the production of sperm. Calcium channel blockers may impair the sperm's ability to penetrate the egg[7]. And high-blood-pressure meds may impair ejaculation. There's a drug for everyone!

Treating Infertility Naturally with Vitamins and Minerals

Probably the most important vitamin for male fertility is vitamin C; probably the most important mineral is zinc.

Vitamin C helps to treat male infertility, especially if the infertility is caused by antibodies against the sperm, which causes the sperm to clump or stick together, an undesirable effect called agglutination. When people stick together, it's a good thing; when sperm stick together, it's not so good. When sperm become agglutinated, your chances of

WHEN PEOPLE STICK TOGETHER, IT'S A GOOD THING; WHEN SPERM STICK TOGETHER... YOUR CHANCES OF FERTILITY DROP OFF.

fertility drop off. But vitamin C reduces agglutination[8]. So, if agglutinated sperm is the problem, try taking the versatile vitamin C.

Vitamin C helps in a number of other ways, too. Sperm is extremely sensitive to free-radical damage, and since vitamin C is an antioxidant, it helps to prevent free-radical damage. Vitamin C is specifically able to protect sperm from that critical enemy. This protective effect of vitamin C is crucial for fertility because free-radical damage can lead to both abnormal sperm and low sperm count.

Vitamin C increases sperm count. In one study, when healthy men decreased their dietary vitamin C from 250 mg a day to 5 mg a day, there was a 91% increase in the number of their sperm with damaged DNA[9]. In another study, infertile men were given 1,000 mg of vitamin C, and after only one week their sperm counts went up by an incredible 140%. After three weeks their sperm count was still going up. Before the start of the study, many of the men had had agglutinated sperm (25% of their sperm was agglutinated: enough to cause infertility), but after three weeks in the study, only 11% of their sperm was agglutinated. After sixty days, all of the men had conceived children with their wives; none of the men in the placebo group had[10].

And there is one more way vitamin C can help. It can help offset the damage that smoking does to sperm quality[11]. So, while it is certainly best to quit smoking, next best is to take vitamin C while you're trying.

Zinc is one of the most crucial nutrients for male sexual function. It is involved with virtually every aspect of male reproduction, and is one of the most essential nutrients in ensuring fertility.

Zinc helps in testosterone production, sperm formation, and motility[12]. A low zinc count is characterized by decreased testosterone. Zinc deficiency also leads to low sperm levels[13] and can atrophy your testicles! So, since seeds and nuts are rich in zinc, it looks like seeds really can build seeds, and nuts really can build . . . well . . . nuts!

So not having enough zinc can be the cause of infertility. And men with infertility typically do have a lower zinc level. But the good news is that adding zinc can improve the underlying problems. If you suffer from infertility, taking zinc supplements can improve sperm count[14], and, according to many, but not all, studies, improve sperm motility[15]. Supplementing zinc can also improve the physical characteristics of sperm[16]; in other words, it can help get them into shape for the hazardous course ahead. Putting them—sperm count, motility, and shape—together, one placebo-controlled study of a hundred men with low sperm motility found that 57 mg of zinc twice a day for three months led to significant improvements in sperm count, motility, and quality. It also led to significant improvements in what it called—sounding more like a gardening study than a human study—"fertilizing capacity"[17].

When researchers looked at thirty-seven men who had actually been infertile for at least five years, they found that those who had low testosterone levels experienced a significant increase in both testosterone levels and sperm count when given 60 mg of zinc for forty-five to fifty days. But the real proof that zinc passed the test is that, even though the study was short, the zinc improved things so much that nine of the twenty-two men who had low testosterone conceived with their partners[18]. All of these results indicate that supplementing zinc is a good idea for men with low sperm counts and motility, especially when testosterone count is low.

In addition to increasing zinc through supplements, you can give it an extra boost by eating lots of whole grains, legumes, seeds, and nuts. If you are using supplements in addition to food, don't go nuts—getting enough zinc is crucial; so is not getting too much. Try around 15 to 30 mg twice a day. If you are taking zinc long-term, add 1 mg of copper for every 10 mg of zinc up to a total of 3 mg to prevent copper deficiency. So, at the dose of zinc we have suggested, add 2 to 3 mg of copper.

Other antioxidants, including vitamin E, selenium, and beta-carotene, also help with male infertility. Vitamin E is the main antioxidant in sperm membranes, where it stops free-radical damage. It appears to carry oxygen to the reproductive organs, helping them to be healthy. It has also been shown to help sperm fertilize eggs in test tubes. Vitamin E is also needed to balance hormone production. Vitamin E has been known as the sex vitamin or the anti-sterility vitamin. Vitamin E's scientific name is tocopherol: tokos is Greek for childbirth or offspring, and phero means to bear. In one preliminary study, 100 to 200 IU of vitamin E given to both partners in infertile couples significantly increased fertility[19].

Supplementing with selenium can also be of aid, since deficiencies of selenium have been linked to reduced sperm counts and sterility. A double-blind study of infertile men with reduced sperm motility found that selenium can increase motility. And 11% of the couples in which the men got selenium conceived compared to 0% who got a placebo[20a].

In the most important antioxidant and fertility research to date, when the highly respected Cochrane group did a review of the research on male infertility and antioxidants, what they found was startlingly impressive. Their review included thirty-four controlled studies that included a total of 2,876 couples who were having difficulties becoming pregnant because the male partner had either low sperm count or low sperm motility. The results showed that when men were given antioxidants, the couples were more than four times more likely to conceive and nearly five times more likely to have a successful delivery. Both improvements were statistically significant, and none of the studies found any evidence of harmful side effects. Vitamin E, zinc, and L-carnitine may have been the most effective[20b].

Vitamin A is also important in reproductive gland function. Another vitamin, vitamin B12, is also needed to stay fertile. Low B12 leads to low sperm count and motility. Supplementing B12 can help with both. Giving B12 increases sperm count in 54% to 60% of men and sperm motility in 50%[21]. In another study, a very large dose of 6 mg of B12 a day was shown to increase sperm count by 37.5%[22]. Even if your B12 is not low, supplementing it can help. When men with normal B12, but with sperm counts less than 20 million per millilitre, took 1,000 mcg of B12, 27% of them increased their count to over 100 million[23].

Another B vitamin, folic acid, though better known for women's health, may also help. Men with mutations in genes that lead to low folate levels are more likely to have trouble fathering children[24], but when 5,000 mcg of folic acid and 66 mg of zinc were given to infertile men, their sperm count nearly doubled[25]. Other B vitamins are also involved in reproductive gland function, so take a B complex.

Treating Infertility Naturally With Amino Acids
Though less well known than the vitamins and minerals, two amino acids are no less important: L-arginine and L-carnitine.

Arginine is very useful in treating infertility in men. It improves both sperm count and motility and also improves sexual desire and ejaculation. Seminal fluid contains arginine, and sexual maturity can be delayed by an arginine deficiency. This amino acid is required for the replication of cells, making it essential for sperm formation. An early study, done over half a century ago, found that after only nine days on an arginine-deficient diet, men's sperm counts dropped by about 90% and the number of non-motile sperm increased nearly tenfold[26].

In one study, L-arginine improved sperm count and motility in a full 74% of men[27]. Several preliminary studies have shown that several months of arginine increases sperm count, quality, and motility, as well as fertility; that is, it has actually been shown to increase your odds of a successful pregnancy[28]. You need to give it several months, as in the studies, because sperm takes about three months to form. The same goes for other nutritional supplements.

Other studies have found no effect of arginine on sperm count. But in these studies, sperm counts were really low. And that seems to be the deciding factor for whether you should try arginine. If sperm count is over 10 million per millilitre, then taking up to 4 g a day is definitely worth trying; if sperm count is under 10 million, save your money and try something else.

The other really important amino acid is L-carnitine. L-carnitine concentrations are extremely high in sperm. This amino acid seems to be crucial for sperm to mature[29], and greater carnitine concentrations correlate with greater number and motility of sperm[30]. Low carnitine levels mean poor sperm development, function, and motility.

Carnitine can improve both sperm count and motility, and the research is impressive, especially on motility. This amino acid provides the energy for the production of sperm and the fuel to drive it.

Sperm quality improves with as little as 1 g of carnitine a day[31]. With improvement in quality comes improvement in motility. So it is not surprising that 2 g of carnitine taken twice a day increases the percentage of motile sperm from 25.5% to 46.7%[32]. In an impressive study, forty-seven men who averaged less than 30% motile sperm—50% or more is normal—were given 3 g of carnitine each day for three months. By the end of the study, an incredible 80% had motility levels close to normal. At least as important, the percentage of sperm that moved forward in a rapid linear motion also increased. These are the sperm that are most likely to succeed: picture a hundred-metre dash where some runners sprint straight to the finish line and some swerve slowly down the course. Carnitine supplementation also increased sperm count in this study[33]. A second study has also found an increase in these "most likely to succeed sperm." When a hundred men with a low percentage of motile sperm were given 3 g of carnitine a day for four months, the sperm with rapid linear motion increased from 10.8% to 18%. Overall motility increased from 26.9% to 37.7% and the sperms' velocity also significantly increased. These sperm were in much improved shape! There were also more of them, with the number of ejaculated sperm increasing significantly[34]. Other research has also found increased count and motility with 3 g of carnitine a day[35].

So can all of this add up to increased pregnancies? The answer seems to be yes. Because when researchers gave 4 g of a form of carnitine known as acetylcarnitine, they found not only significant increases in the all-important percentage of sperm with rapid linear motion, but also that 35% of the female partners became pregnant[36].

Treating Infertility Naturally with Herbs and Other Supplements

Some herbs may also help. Ginseng is used to restore vitality and energy, and, according to herbalist Rosemary Gladstar, is especially good for building sexual vitality. Ginseng increases mental and physical performance and combats stress—all important factors when you are trying to conceive. Ginseng has been shown to produce a rise in sperm count, motility, and testosterone, suggesting it has an important role in treating infertility in addition to its important role in treating impotence[37].

Siberian ginseng, now known as eleuthero, has also been used to increase reproductive capacity and sperm count, and has an ancient tradition as a stimulant of male virility. It is used to combat fatigue and stress and to provide energy and vitality.

The excellent immune and tonifying herb, astragalus, has been shown in one study to significantly stimulate sperm motility[38]. It is especially valuable if infection is present.

INFECTION BUSTERS: HERBS AND SUPPLEMENTS THAT REDUCE INFECTIONS WHICH CAN CAUSE INFERTILITY

ASTRAGALUS
FLOWER POLLEN
GARLIC
GOLDENSEAL
ECHINACEA
BUCHU
CORN SILK
UVA URSI
WILD INDIGO
MYRRH
BROMELAIN

Flower pollen can also work to reduce infection that can cause infertility.

Other immune helpers that can help to get rid of infection include garlic, goldenseal, Echinacea, buchu, corn silk, uva ursi, wild indigo, and myrrh. Bromelain can also help. Infection in the prostate in men or urinary tract in men and women can cause infertility.

Rhodiola can also help to improve stress and men's sexual reproductive health.

Goji berries have been used traditionally to increase sperm production, and one double-blind study found that the herb increased "sexual activity," though we were not able to ascertain specifically what "activity" was increased[39].

The mysterious maca, now familiar to you from the chapters on impotence and on folklore, potions, and aphrodisiacs, makes yet another appearance for infertility. This little-known herb seems to be everywhere, and it is still to make one more appearance later in this book. In a very small and uncontrolled study—so be cautious before you get too excited—1.5 g and 3 g a day of maca improved sperm production and motility without affecting hormones[40].

The remarkable Chinese herb ho shou wu, also known as fo ti, has been traditionally used to build sperm.

Studies have also shown that Pycnogenol®, the antioxidant-rich extract from pine bark, may improve sperm quality and function. And preliminary research has found that SAMe, a very important nutrient for depression, osteoarthritis, fibromyalgia, migraines, and liver problems, but not usually thought of for infertility, may increase sperm activity in infertile men when taken at a dose of 800 mcg a day.

Several studies have also shown that acupuncture improves poor sperm function[41].

Treating Infertility Naturally with Diet
Helpful foods for treating the male sexual system include nuts and seeds, since they are high in zinc, essential fatty acids (essential for normal glandular

functioning and activity in the reproductive system), fibre, and other nutrients. If estrogen is high or testosterone is low, soy foods can be helpful since they are rich in phytoestrogens, which can lower estrogen when it is too high, and their phytosterols, which are similar to testosterone, may be used by the body to produce hormones. If testosterone is low, in addition to soy beans, eat lots of other beans as well as nuts and seeds. Make sure your diet is high in fibre. For those who do not have candida, yeast is also a good food to use.

As we saw with female infertility, the types of fats you eat can play an important role, and in male infertility, as in all other aspects of health, the good guys and the bad guys are the same old fats. Infertile men should avoid saturated fats and increase polyunsaturated fats. Saturated fats are found in animal products such as butter, lard, meat, and dairy products. Polyunsaturated fats improve sperm formation and activity. And stay away from trans fatty acids: they can contribute to abnormal sperm. Michael T. Murray, N.D., says that you should also avoid cottonseed oil, which contains gossypol, a substance that has been shown in studies to reduce sperm count[42]. He also says to avoid shortening, hydrogenated margarine, and coconut and palm oil, because these oils contain hydrogenated oils or saturated oils that are bad for fertility. Increase EFAs such as flaxseed oil, hemp oil, and polyunsaturated oils from nuts and seeds; these oils can help in all aspects of sexual function.

And finally, eating organically may help. One study found surprisingly high sperm counts in organic farmers. Their sperm count was more than double that of a control group, suggesting that eating organic food may increase fertility[43].

TREATMENT SUMMARY
Diet & Lifestyle
- Eat lots of nuts and seeds, soy and other beans
- Increase polyunsaturated essential fatty acids; avoid saturated fats and trans fats
- Make as much of your food as possible organic
- Reduce alcohol
- Quit smoking
- Avoid estrogen-mimicking chemicals in pesticide and plastic

- Attain a healthy weight
- Avoid hot tubs, saunas, and tight-fitting pants
- Acupuncture

Nutritional Supplements
- Vitamin C: at least 1,000mg
- Zinc: 15-30mg twice a day
- Vitamin E: 200-800IU
- Folic acid: 400-5,000mcg
- Arginine: up to 4g a day if sperm count is over 10 million per millilitre
- L-carnitine: 3-4g a day

Herbs
- Ginseng: 1-3g
- Astragalus (especially if there is an infection): 1-1.5g three times a day or 2-6ml tincture three times a day
- Rhodiola rosea, goji berry, maca and ho shou wu may also help

ENDNOTES

1. Sallmen, M., *et al*. Reduced fertility among overweight and obese men. *Epidemiology* 2006; 17:520–23.

2. Field, B., M. Selub, C. L. Hughes. Reproductive effects of environmental agents. *Semin Rep Endocrinol* 1990; 8:44–55; Sharpe, R. M., N. E. Skakkebaek. Are oestrogens involved in falling sperm counts and disorders of the male reproductive tract? *Lancet* 1993; 341:1392–95.

3. Carlsen, E., *et al*. Decline in semen quality from 1930 to 1991. *Ugeskr Laeger* 1993; 155:2530–35.

4. Carlsen, E., *et al*. Evidence for decreasing quality of semen during past 50 years. *Br Med J* 1992; 305:609–13; Carlsen, E., *et al*. Decline in semen quality from 1930 to 1991. *Ugeskr Laeger* 1993; 155:2530–35.

5. Kulikauskas, V. D., D. Blaustein, D. Ablin. Cigarette smoking and its possible effects on sperm. *Fertil Steril* 1985; 44:526–28; Hruska, K. S., *et al*. Environmental factors in infertility. *Clin Obstet Gynecol* 2000; 43:821–29; Zhang, J. P., *et al*. Effect of smoking on semen quality of infertile men in Shandong, China. *Asian J Androl* 2000; 2:143–46; Wang, S. L., *et al*. A study on occupational exposure to petrochemicals and smoking on seminal quality. *J Androl* 2001; 22:73–78.

6. Goverde, H. J. M., *et al*. Semen quality and frequency of smoking and alcohol consumption—an explorative study. *Int J Fertil* 1995; 40:135–38.

7. Katsoff, D., J. H. Check. A challenge to the concept that the use of calcium channel blockers causes reversible male infertility. *Hum Reprod* 1997; 12:1480–82.

8. Dawson, E. B., W. A. Harris, W. J. McGanity. Effect of ascorbic acid on sperm fertility. *Fed Proc* 1983; 42:531; Dawson, E., *et al*. Effect of ascorbic acid on male fertility. *Ann NY Acad Sci* 1987; 498:312–23.

9. Fraga, C., *et al*. Ascorbic acid protects against endogenous oxidative DNA

damage in human sperm. *Proc Natl Acad Sci* 1991; 88:11003–006.

10. Dawson, E., *et al*. Effect of ascorbic acid on male fertility. *Ann NY Acad Sci* 1987; 498:312–23.

11. Dawson, E., W. Harris, L. Powell. Effect of vitamin C supplementation on sperm quality of heavy smokers. *FASEB J* 1991; 5:A915; Dawson, E. B., *et al*. Effect of ascorbic acid supplementation on the sperm quality of smokers. *Fertil Steril* 1992; 58:1034–39.

12. Prasad, A. S. Zinc in growth and development and spectrum of human zinc deficiency. *J Am Coll Nutr* 1988; 7:377–84.

13. Prasad, A. S., Z. T. Cossack. Zinc supplementation and growth in sickle cell disease. *Ann Intern Med* 1984; 100:367–71.

14. Stankovic, H., D. Mikac-Devic. Zinc and copper in human semen. *Clin Chim Acta* 1976; 70:123–26; Hartoma, T. R., K. Nahoul, A. Netter. Zinc, plasma androgens and male sterility. *Lancet* 1977; 2:1125–26.

15. Stankovic, H., D. Mikac-Devic. Zinc and copper in human semen. *Clin Chim Acta* 1976; 70:123–26; Kynaston, H. G., *et al*. Changes in seminal quality following oral zinc therapy. *Andrologia* 1988; 20:21–22.

16. Tikkiwal, M., R. L. Ajmera, N. K. Mathur. Effect of zinc administration on seminal zinc and fertility of oligospermic males. *Indian J Physiol Pharmacol* 1987; 31:30–34.

17. Omu, A. E., H. Dashti, S. Al-Othman. Treatment of asthenozoospermia with zinc sulphate: andrological, immunological and obstetric outcome. *Eur J Obstet Gynecol Reprod Biol* 1998; 79:179–84.

18. Netter, A., *et al*. Effect of zinc administration on plasma testosterone, dihydrotestosterone and sperm count. *Arch Androl* 1982; 7:69–73.

19. Bayer, R. Treatment of infertility with vitamin E. *Int J Fertil* 1960; 5:70–78.

20a. Scott, R., *et al.* The effect of oral selenium supplementation on human sperm motility. *Br J Urol* 1998; 82:76–80.

20b. Showell, M. G., *et al.* Antioxidants for male subfertility. *Cochrane Database of Syst Rev* 2011;1:CD007411. DOI: 10.1002/14651858.CD007411. pub2.

21. Isoyama, R., *et al.* Clinical experience with methylcobalamin (CH3–B12) for male infertility. *Hinyokika Kiyo* 1984; 30:581–86; Isoyama, R., *et al.* Clinical experience of methyl-cobalamin (CH3–B12)/clomiphene citrate combined treatment in male infertility. *Hinyokika Kiyo* 1986; 32:1177–83.

22. Moriyama, H., *et al.* Studies on the usefulness of a long-term, high-dose treatment of methylcobalamin in patients with oligozoospermia. *Hinyokika Kiyo* 1987; 33:151–56.

23. Sandler, B., B. Faragher. Treatment of oligospermia with vitamin B12. *Infertility* 1984; 7:133–38.

24. Besold, G., M. Lange, R. U. Peter. Homozygous methylenetetra-hydrofolate reductase C677T mutation and male fertility. *N Engl J Med* 2001; 344:1172–73; Lee, H. C., *et al.* Association study of four polymorphisms in three folate-related enzyme genes with non-obstructive male infertility. *Human Reproduction* 2006; 21:3162–70.

25. Wong, W.Y., *et al.* Effects of folic acid and zinc sulfate on male factor subfertility: A double-blind, randomized, placebo-controlled trial. *Fertility and Sterility* 2002; 77:491–98.

26. Holt, L. E., Jr., A. A. Albanesse. Observations on amino acid deficiencies in men. *Trans Assoc Am Physicians* 1944; 58:143–56.

27. Schacter, A., J. A. Goldman, Z. Zukerman. Treatment of oligospermia with the amino acid arginine. *J Urol* 1973; 110:311–13.

28. Tanimura, J. Studies on arginine in human semen. Part II. The effects of

medication with L-arginine-HCl on male infertility. *Bull Osaka Med School* 1967; 13:84–89; Schacter, A., *et al.* Treatment of oligospermia with the amino acid arginine. *Int J Gynaecol Obstet* 1973; 11:206–09; De Aloysio, D., *et al.* The clinical use of arginine aspartate in male infertility. *Acta Eur Fertil* 1982; 13:133–67; Scibona, M., *et al.* L-arginine and male infertility. *Minerva Urol Nefrol* 1994; 46:251–53.

29. Golan, R., *et al.* Influences of various substrates on the acetylcarnitine: carnitine ratio in motile and immotile human spermatozoa. *Reprod Fert* 1986; 78:287–93.

30. Menchini-Fabris, G. F., *et al.* Free L-carnitine in human semen: its variability in different andrologic pathologies. *Fertil Steril* 1984; 42:263–67.

31. Müller-Tyl, E., *et al.* Wirkung von carnitin auf spermienzahl und spermien motilität. *Fertilität* 4:1–4; Loumbakis, P., *et al.* Effects of L-carnitine in patients with asthenospermia. *Eur J Urol* 30(suppl 2):954.

32. Campaniello, E., *et al.* Carnitine administration in asthenopspermia. IV International Congress of Andrology, Firenze, May 14–18.

33. Vitali, G., R. Parente, C. Melotti. Carnitine supplementation in human idiopathic asthenospermia: clinical results. *Drugs Exptl Clin Res* 1995; 21:157–59.

34. Costa, M., *et al.* L-carnitine in idiopathic asthenozoospermia: a multicenter study. *Andologia* 1994; 26:155–59.

35. Micic, S. effects of L-carnitine on sperm motility and number in infertile men. 16th World Congress on Fert Steril, and 54th Annual Meeting of the Am Soc reprod Med, San Francisco, Oct 4–9, 1998.

36. Moncada, M. L., *et al.* Effects of acetylcarnitine treatment in oligoasthenospermia patients. *Acta Europaea Fertilitatis* 1992; 23:221–24.

37. Salvati, G., *et al.* Effects of *Panax ginseng* C.A. Meyer saponins on male

fertility. *Panmineva Med* 1996; 38:249–54.

38. Hong, C.Y., J. Ku, P. Wu. *Astragalus membranaceus* stimulates human sperm motility *in vitro. Am J Chin Med* 1992; 20:289–94.

39. Amagase, H., D. M. Nance. A. randomized, double-blind, placebo-controlled, clinical study of the general effects of a standardized *Lycium barbarum* (goji) juice, GoChi™. *J Altern Complement Med* 2008; 14: 403–412.

40. Gonzales, G. F., *et al. Lepidium meyenii* (maca) improves semen parameters in adult men. *Asian J Androl* 2001; 3:301–03.

41. Riegler, R., *et al.* Correlation of psychological changes and spermiogram improvements following acupuncture. *Urologe [A]* 1984; 23:329–33; Fischl, F., *et al.* Modification of semen quality by acupuncture in subfertile males. *Geburtshilfe Fraunheilkd* 1984; 44:510–12; Siterman, S., *et al.* Effect of acupuncture on sperm parameters of males suffering from subfertility related to low sperm quality. *Arch Androl* 1997; 39:155–61.

42. Weller, D. P., L. J. D. Zaneveld, N. R. Farnsworth. Gossypol: Pharmacology and current status as a male contraceptive. *Econ Med Plant Red* 1985; 1:87–112.

43. Abell, A., E. Ernst, J. P. Bonde. High sperm density among members of organic farmers' association. *Lancet* 1994; 343:1498.

Part III

Conditions that Contribute to the Big Three and Interfere with the Enjoyment of Sexuality

Chapter Five

ACHIEVING A HEALTHY WEIGHT

A chapter on weight loss is included in this book for one important reason. Not because we are endorsing the modern trend toward skinny at all cost. Not because of superficial connections between body appearance and sexuality. And not to promote any fad diets, which are invariably unhealthy and ineffective in the long run.

We have included it for one reason only—because obesity showed up as a major inhibitor of healthy reproduction in each of the female infertility, male infertility, and erectile dysfunction chapters. Keep in mind that the change in weight often does not need to be dramatic; fertility is very sensitive to weight change. Keep in mind, too, that the weight loss needs to be not only effective, but healthy; you are priming your body for creating another life.

In the past several years, all kinds of weight-loss diets have emerged. And many of them have made a lot of money for a lot of people. But many of them, while hooking you in in the short run, are ineffective in the long run; many are not good for you and some are downright crazy and dangerous. Though most diets will lead to weight loss in the short term—following almost any controlled diet will be better than the out-of-control diet many of us follow—the really hard part is maintaining the weight loss. And there is virtually no research proving which, if any, of these diets is actually effective for the long-term weight loss that leads to real improvements in health. Just as disturbing, there is scant research on the long-term healthfulness of these weight-loss diets. So it would be crucially important to know which weight-loss diets and supplements really increase our chances of maintaining a healthy weight and which ones are really healthy for us to use.

Which Diet Really Keeps Weight Off?

In one of the few, and perhaps the only, studies to look at long-term, sustainable weight loss, sixty-four overweight women were put on either a low-fat diet or a vegan diet. Vegan diets exclude all animal products, and the one used in this study also limited nuts, seeds, and avocados. The women on the vegan diet lost significantly more weight. After a year, the vegans had lost eleven pounds compared to only four in the low-fat group, and they were still seven pounds lighter after two years, while the women in the low-fat group were only two pounds lighter[1]. So the vegan diet just might be the first one to have proven itself effective over the long run.

These researchers probably restricted nuts, seeds, and avocados because of the common conception that they are fattening. But the restriction was unnecessary. Studies consistently show that, despite the difficult-to-shake reputation, nuts are not fattening and are great for your heart. Women who eat a handful of raw unsalted nuts a day are more likely to be a healthy weight. Various nuts have been shown in various studies to lower the heart-damaging LDL cholesterol while raising the heart-healthy HDL cholesterol without increasing weight[2]. Nuts have also been shown to reduce your risk of dying from heart disease[3]. Similarly, recent research has also acquitted the avocado from charges of being fattening.

Which Diets Are Healthy for You?

The good news is that the same sort of diet that really works is the same sort of diet that is really good for you. The bonus is that this diet is also completely consistent with the research on diet and fertility that we saw in the earlier chapters.

A new study has finally compared how good for you the different weight-loss diets are. And it turns out the popular low-carb diets are the worst, while the high-complex-carb ones are the best.

Which one is the very healthiest? Dean Ornish's plan takes first place. His diet is a vegetarian diet that is high in fibre and complex carbs and very low in cholesterol and saturated fat. The second best is the Weight Watcher's high-carb (but not the low-carb) version. The unhealthiest of all is the low-carb Atkins diet[4].

So you want to lose weight and maintain it in a way that is safe and healthy for you? Science says eat a vegetarian/vegan diet that is high in fibre and complex carbs from legumes, whole grains, fruits, and vegetables and very low in animal fats and proteins. And go ahead and throw in the nuts and seeds.

Linda's Fifteen Tips for Healthy Weight Loss[5]

- Drink eight glasses of water a day.
- Eat plenty of fibre every day.
- Eat vegetables (juice/salad) at the beginning of meals to load you up with healthy, non-fattening nutrients and to fill you up faster.
- Eat vegetables and fruits for snacks.
- After meals, swish your mouth or brush your teeth right away. This signals your brain that the meal is over.
- Use apple cider vinegar in salad dressings.
- Don't skip meals: it will slow your metabolism down, and it will make you overeat at the next meal.
- Overeating and eating sweets is often masking a desire for affection or love. So get a hug instead, or give one. Kiss your cat or dog. Better yet, take your dog for a walk.
- Don't eat in front of the TV: it causes overeating.
- Drink water when you first begin to feel hungry: thirst signals can be confused as hunger signals, which lead to overeating.
- Don't eat when you are bored. Ask yourself, "Am I really hungry?"
- Put small portions on your plate. You can take more if needed, but studies show that if you put larger amounts of food on your plate you

will overeat.

- Eat with someone: you are less likely to overeat.
- Keep healthy snacks washed and ready to go, cut up in the fridge. Try celery sticks, cucumber, berries, radishes, grapefruit, pineapple, mango, and peppers.
- Walk for an hour every day. Make this part of your lifestyle. It will keep the weight off, the stress down, and keep you feeling energized and stimulated, and less in need of a binge. Find a friend to walk with you; it helps. For me, it is often the best part of my day.

Which Supplements Really Work?

Fibre: Filling Up and Controlling Blood Sugar

From the studies on which diets really work and which diets are really safe, it should now not be a surprise that fibre really helps. A review of studies found that, even when you don't restrict calories, high-fibre diets improve weight loss[6]. Fibre makes you feel full, so you eat less[7]. But it does more than that. Fibre helps control blood sugar and insulin, and blood sugar and insulin control is crucial for weight control. Psyllium, pectin, guar gum, and glucomannan are especially good fibre supplements for weight loss. People given 3 g of glucomannan a day for two months have been shown to lose between 5.5 and 8.14 pounds, while people given a placebo continued to gain weight[8]. Other studies also testify to the weight-loss power of glucomannan[9].

5-HTP: The Undiscovered Secret

5-hydroxytryptophan, or 5-HTP for short, is a compound extracted from plants and turned into a supplement that raises serotonin. That's why it's one of the best nutrients for depression and insomnia. But less known is that serotonin signals your brain that you are full and should stop eating. So if your serotonin is low, your brain thinks you're hungry and sends out a red alert for food. You start craving the fastest possible energy source and binge on sugary and refined foods. So serotonin deficiency is a big contributor to weight gain.

5-HTP corrects the deficiency. When obese women were given 200 mg of 5-HTP three times a day, twenty minutes before meals, their calorie intake went down by 37%, and they lost three pounds in five weeks even though they were not exercising and were allowed to eat whatever they wanted. A placebo-control group lost only one pound[10].

Two other weight-loss studies gave either 5-HTP or a placebo to obese women half an hour before each meal. In the first, the placebo group lost 2.28 pounds in six weeks and the 5-HTP group lost 10.34[11]. In the second, the placebo group lost 1.87 pounds in twelve weeks, while the 5-HTP group lost 11.63 pounds[12]. Those are impressive numbers!

Though no studies have suggested that 5-HTP is harmful during pregnancy—because its safety for pregnant women is not yet established—if you are using it as an aid for weight loss to help enhance fertility, to be safe, you should stop taking it if you think there is a chance you have conceived.

Other ways of increasing serotonin include using SAMe and St. John's wort.

Hydroxycitrate: Eat Less; Make Less Fat

From the fruit of the Malabar tamarind (*Garcinia cambogia*) comes hydroxycitrate. Hydroxycitrate inhibits appetite, so fewer calories go in, and inhibits fat production from carbohydrates, so fewer of those calories become fat. Though there has been one negative study, several preliminary studies suggest that hydroxycitrate is a powerful inhibitor of fat production. A recent double-blind study found that this herb significantly improves results of weight loss diets[13]. Canadian herbalist Terry Willard, Ph.D., says that he has seen people get very good results using this herb.

Green Tea: Drink the Pounds Away

A very healthy, effective, inexpensive, and delicious way to lose weight is green tea. Green tea helps weight loss by stimulating thermogenesis[14]. Thermogenic substances turn up the body heat and literally burn the calories away. Green tea especially targets weight loss in the waist, which is important because losing weight in the abdominal area may be the most important kind of weight loss for living longer. Obese women who were given 250 mg of powdered green tea eight times a day in a double-blind, placebo-controlled study, lost 1.9 kg in thirty days and significantly decreased their waist measurement[15]. Another study produced a 4.6% decrease in weight and a 4.5% decrease in waist size[16]. Most recently, overweight men and women who did not exercise were put on an exercise program and given either green tea that had its catechin content enriched

or a placebo beverage. Abdominal fat went down by 7.7% in the green tea group and only by 4.4% in the placebo group[17]. Drink your green tea regularly; it's delicious and a great source of healthy antioxidants, too. An added bonus if you are trying to lose weight to address polycystic ovary syndrome and increase your chances of fertility is that green tea may specifically help with that goal (see female infertility chapter).

To boost thermogenesis, you can also try an old herbal formula, using such herbs as cayenne powder and/or ginger powder mixed with hot water and, if you like, apple cider vinegar. This formula helps to turn up your body's heat and burn fat. Modern research has validated the traditional belief about cayenne: studies confirm that it does reduce calories consumed and increase calories burned[18].

Burn the Calories Away

Another herb that increases the amount of calories you burn through thermogenesis is *citrus aurantium*, or bitter orange[19]. Citrus aurantium also helps by building lean muscle and making fat available for energy. You probably should not combine this herb with caffeine, though.

Here's a New One: 7-Keto

The supplement 7-keto, that comes from the adrenal hormone DHEA, up-regulates metabolism and stimulates thermogenesis. Double-blind research found that when either 100 mg of 7-keto or a placebo was given twice a day to people who were exercising and controlling their calories, only the 7-keto group lost a significant amount of weight: 6.34 pounds in eight weeks[20].

Chromium: Lose Weight and Build Muscle

Chromium is necessary in the metabolism of carbohydrates, proteins, and fats. It is also a key factor in balancing your sugar levels. Studies have shown that chromium can lower body weight while it increases lean body mass and muscle, probably by increasing your body's sensitivity to insulin[21]. According to Michael Murray, N.D., "Improving insulin sensitivity is an important goal in a weight loss program. Loss of insulin sensitivity is the hallmark feature of obesity. Chromium is a trace mineral necessary for the proper action of insulin on blood sugar control"[22].

One study revealed that people taking chromium lost an average of seven times more body fat than those taking a placebo[23]. Not all weight-loss studies on chromium have been as positive, but a review of double-blind studies concluded that chromium has a small but beneficial effect on weight loss[24]. Most North Americans are deficient in chromium, so supplementation with chromium is very important.

Lose the Liquid, Lose the Weight

Coenzyme Q10 is a powerful antioxidant that can help you lose weight in two ways: by getting rid of excess fluid in your body and by increasing energy through feeding the ATP cycle—your body's energy source. As many as 50% of overweight people are deficient in CoQ10. Another way to get rid of excess water is to take 50 mg of B6 three times per day, and/or dandelion leaf.

Lipotropic Factors

Lipotropic substances, such as choline, inositol, methionine, and betaine, essentially help get the excess fat out of the body. The liver is responsible for breaking down fat, but this ability is reduced in many people. Lipotropics can help improve this function. They enhance the decongestion of the liver, thus improving liver function and encouraging fat metabolism, helping you to lose weight. Like green tea, the inositol may pull double duty since it can also lead to more weight loss and more periods in women with polycystic ovary disease (see female infertility chapter).

Carnitine: Making Energy, not Fat

Carnitine can help weight loss by transporting fat into body cells where it can be burned as energy instead of being stored as fat. Here's one that does double duty for guys (see male infertility chapter).

Sea Vegetables

Sea vegetables such as kelp, nori, dulse, wakame, and hijiki are best known for their ability to affect an under-active thyroid—a cause of weight gain—positively. The iodine in sea vegetables helps to correct an under-active thyroid and encourages metabolic activity. Iodine assists in making thyroid hormones, which are necessary for maintaining normal metabolism.

Balancing Hormones and Losing Weight

Here's an interesting fact: estrogen levels that are too high can actually cause weight gain. The more unnecessary estrogen you have, the harder it can be to lose weight. So try the herb chastetree berry to help you rebalance too high estrogen levels and lose weight. And conveniently, chastetree berry, once again, will help increase fertility while decreasing weight (see female infertility chapter).

Calcium: Building Bone, Losing Weight?

Could weight loss be a new use for calcium? If your diet is low in calcium, it could be. In a huge, seven-year-long double-blind study of 36,282 post-menopausal women, those who got less than 1,200 mg of calcium a day going into the study were less likely to gain weight when given 1,000 mg of supplemental calcium and 400 IU of vitamin D than when they were given a placebo[25]. In a second study, people on a low-calorie diet lost significantly more weight when they were given 800 mg of calcium than when they were given a placebo[26].

Spice Up Your Food

And finally, as mentioned, cayenne may reduce your hunger and calorie consumption, while increasing your calorie burning. So use it liberally in your cooking along with other hot nutrients like ginger and hot peppers.

And slow down and enjoy your meal. You're twice as likely to be overweight if you eat quickly or if you eat until you're full. You're more than three times as likely to be overweight if you do both[27].

Remember that being too thin can cause infertility, too, so the goal is to achieve a healthy weight; the diet still needs to be healthy and full of nutrients because you are preparing yourself for pregnancy.

TREATMENT SUMMARY

Diet & Lifestyle
- Vegetarian diet
- Drink plenty of water
- Exercise

Nutritional Supplements

Choose one or a combination of:
- 5-HTP: 100-200mg three times a day (do not use 5-HTP if you are pregnant)
- Chromium: 200-400mcg
- Coenzyme Q10: 100-300mg

Herbs
- Hydroxycitrate: 500mg three times a day
- Citrus aurantium: 4-6g a day; 320mg, standardized for 4% total alkaloids, five times a day
- Drink green tea or take 2,000mg powdered green tea in several broken doses
- Chastetree berry if your estrogen is too high
- You can also try lipotropic factors, carnitine and seaweed

ENDNOTES

1. Turner-McGrievy, G. M., N. D. Barnard, A. R. Scialli. A two-year randomized weight-loss trial comparing a vegan diet to a more moderate low-fat diet. *Obesity* 2007; 15:2276–81.

2. Rogelio, U. A., *et al.* Effects of walnut consumption on plasma fatty acids and lipoproteins in combined hyperlipidemia. *Am J Clin Nutr* 2001; 74:72–79; Garg, M. L., R. J. Blake, R. B. H. Wills. Macadamia nut consumption lowers plasma total and LDL cholesterol levels in hypercholesterolemic men. *Journal of Nutrition* 2003; 133:1060–63; Jambazian, P. R., *et al.* Almonds in the diet simultaneously improve plasma alpha- tocopherol concentrations and reduce plasma lipids. *J Am Dietetic Association* 2005; 105:449–54.

3. Christine, M., *et al.* Nut consumption and decreased risk of sudden cardiac death in the physicians' health study. *Arch Intern Med* 2002; 162:1382–87.

4. Ma, Y., *et al.* A dietary quality comparison of popular weight-loss plans. *J Am Diet Assoc* 2007; 107:1701.

5. From Linda Woolven, *Smart Woman's Guide to PMS and Pain-free Periods*. Mississauga, ON: John Wiley & Sons, 2008.

6. Howarth, N. C., E. Saltzman, S. B. Roberts. Dietary fiber and weight regulation. *Nutr Rev* 2001; 59:129–39.

7. Burton-Freeman, B. Dietary fiber and energy regulation. *J Nutr* 2000; 130(2S Suppl):272S–275S.

8. Walsh, D. E., V. Yaghoubian, A. Behforooz. Effect of glucomannan on obese patients: a clinical study. *Int J Obes* 1984; 8:289–93; Biancardi, G., L. Palmiero, P. E. Ghirardi. Glucomannan in the treatment of overweight patients with osteoarthritis. *Curr Ther Res* 1989; 46:908–12.

9. Vita, P. M., *et al.* Chronic use of glucomannan in the dietary treatment of severe obesity. *Minerva Med* 1992; 83:135–39; Livieri, C., F. Novazi, R. Lorini. The use of highly purified glucomannan-based fibers in childhood obesity. *Pediatr Med Chir* 1992; 14:195–8.

10. Ceci, F., *et al.* The effects of oral 5-hydroxytryptophan administration on feeding behavior in obese adult female subjects. *Journal of Neural Transmission* 1989; 76:109–17.

11. Cangiano, C., *et al.* Effects of 5-hydoxytryptophan on eating behavior and adherence to dietary prescriptions in obese adult subjects. *Adv Exp Med Biol* 1991; 294:591–93.

12. Cangiano, C., *et al.* Eating behavior and adherence to dietary prescriptions in obese adult subjects treated with 5-hydroxytryptophan. *Am J Clin Nutr* 1992; 56:863–67.

13. Mattes, R. D., L. Bormann. Effects of (-)-hydroxycitric acid on appetitive variables. *Physiol Behav* 2000; 71:87–94.

14. Dulloo, A. G., *et al.* Efficacy of green tea extract rich in catechin polyphenols and caffeine in increasing 24-h energy expenditure and fat oxidation in humans. *Am J Clin Nutr* 1999; 70:1040–45.

15. Lecomte, A. Green tea 'Arkocaps' / Phytotrim® double-blind clinical results. *Revue De L'assoc Mondiale de Phytother* 1985; 1:36–40.

16. Chantre, P., D. Lairon. Recent findings of green tea extract AR25 (Exolise) and its activity for the treatment of obesity. *Phytomedicine* 2002; 9:3–8.

17. Maki, K. C., *et al.* Green Tea Catechin Consumption Enhances Exercise-Induced Abdominal Fat Loss in Overweight and Obese Adults. *J Nutr* 2009; 2:264–70.

18. Henry, C., B. Emery. Effect of spiced food on metabolic rate. *Human Nutr Clin Nutr* 1986; 40:165–8; Yoshioka, M., *et al.* Effects of red-pepper diet on the energy metabolism in men. *J Nutr Sci Vitaminol (Tokyo)* 1995; 41:647–56; Yoshioka, M., *et al.* Effects of red pepper added to high-fat and high-carbohydrate meals on energy metabolism and substrate utilization in Japanese women. *Br J Nutr* 1998; 80:503–10; Yoshioka, M., *et al.* Effects of red pepper on appetite and energy intake. *Br J Nutr* 1999; 82:115–23.

19. Gougeon, R., *et al.* Increase in the thermic effect of food in women by adrenergic amines extracted from citrus aurantium. *Obes Res* 2005; 13:1187–94.

20. Kalman, D. S., *et al.* A randomized, double-blind, placebo controlled study of 3-acetyl-7-oxo-dehydroepiandrosterone in healthy overweight adults. *Curr Ther Res* 2000; 61:435–42.

21. McCarthy, M. F. Hypothesis: Sensitization of insulin-dependent hypothalamic glucoreceptors may account for the fat-reducing effects of chromium picolinate. *J Optimal Nutr* 1993; 21:36–53; Crawford, V., R. Scheckenbach, H. G. Preuss. Effects of niacin-bound chromium supplementation on body composition in overweight African-American women. *Diabetes Obes Metab* 1999; 1:331–37.

22. Murray, M. T. *Natural Alternatives for Weight Loss.* New York, NY: William Morrow and Company, 1996.

23. Evans, G. W., D. J. Pouchnik. Composition and biological activity of chromium-pyridine cabosylate complexes. *J Inorganic Biochemistry* 1993; 49:177–87.

24. Pittler, M. H., C. Stevinson, E. Ernst. Chromium picolinate for reducing body weight: meta-analysis of randomized trials. *Int J Obes Relat Metab Disord* 2003; 27:522–29.

25. Caan, B., *et al.* Calcium plus vitamin D supplementation and the risk of postmenopausal weight gain. *Arch Intern Med* 2007; 167:893–902.

26. Zemel, M. B., *et al.* Calcium and dairy acceleration of weight and fat loss during energy restriction in obese adults. *Obes Res* 2004; 12:582–90.

27. Maruyama, K. *et al.* The joint impact of self-reported behaviours of eating quickly and eating until full on overweight: results of a cross-sectional survey. *BMJ* 2008; 337:a2002.

Chapter Six

RESTORING VITALITY AFTER BIRTH: POSTPARTUM DEPRESSION AND LOW LIBIDO

For many women, the time after birth can be one of low energy, depleted stores, and, for some, depression, anxiety, and loss of libido. These problems can be caused by hormone levels that might have dropped very low in the first year after birth and by thyroid levels that might be out of whack. Lack of sleep can also contribute, because you are getting up to breast-feed your baby at night. Of course, low energy and depression are not going to lead to a desire for sex. Also, many women are sore or feel unattractive after birth, and their minds are simply on the new life they've just brought into the world. So some time may be needed to heal properly and to regain some strength before returning to sex. Adjustments need to be made to help incorporate this new life into the woman's life. Time is needed to exercise and eat right to feel like your old self again.

Herbs that Bring You Calm
But what can you do to help restore yourself and get back to normal? Start by using gentle, mild herbal nervines as teas to help you relax and get calm and get the sleep you need. Try skullcap, lemon balm, valerian, motherwort, chamomile, and lavender.

You should also consider herbs that help to provide extra nourishment, like red raspberry leaf, which is also used for postpartum depression, nettle, oat straw, seaweeds such as kelp, dulse, and nori, and deep green leafy vegetables, for extra nutrition. A tea made from burdock root could help your body get its strength back.

Vitamins and Minerals that Bring You Back

And don't forget calcium and magnesium for stress and anxiety and sleeplessness. A good-quality multivitamin, with B-vitamins, will also help to replenish depleted stores and help fight depression and low libido. Low B6, folic acid, and low B vitamins in general can cause nerve instability and depression; they may even lower serotonin, a key neurotransmitter for maintaining mood stability. So take a B-complex. Evening primrose oil might help to restore mood after a delivery, so try taking two 500-mg capsules two times a day for six to eight weeks. Flaxseed oil may also help. Low iron or low potassium can also cause depression, another reason to take a good-quality multivitamin/mineral compound.

Diet that Defeats Depression

And be sure to eat well. Make sure your diet is high in fibre and rich in nutrients. Not enough of the healthy dietary fats or too much of the wrong fats is linked to postpartum depression, so be sure to eat a well-balanced diet (see chapter on women's fertility for information on healthy and unhealthy fats). Eat a whole-food diet that focuses on vegetables of different colours, whole grains, fruits, legumes, and raw seeds and nuts. Avoid refined foods and chemicals. Drinking coffee is also linked to depression, so cut the caffeine. It's a good idea to try cutting all sources of caffeine, including black tea, chocolate, and soft drinks.

Antidepressant Herbal Tea

For depression, which can lead to lack of libido, try Rosemary Gladstar's herbal "Joy Tea":

- 2 parts chamomile
- 3 parts lemon balm
- 1 part hawthorn berries and blossoms

- 2 parts hibiscus
- 2 parts rose petals
- 1/8 part lavender flowers
- 1/8 part cardamom pods, chopped

Use 4 to 6 tablespoons of herbs per quart of water. Add herbs to cold water and place in direct sunlight. Let sit for several hours or overnight. Strain and enjoy. Use fresh herbs and flowers.

You can also try placing a bowl of fresh-scented blossoms such as rose, lavender, and borage flowers, in the room. And diffuse the air with the essential oil bergamot for depression and with lavender essential oil for anxiety.

Antidepressant Herbs and Nutrients

Red raspberry leaf tea is fantastic for a depression that can cause low libido. Or try St. John's wort, 5-HTP, and/or SAMe. SAMe has been shown to be of benefit in postpartum depression. In a study of postpartum depression, women taking 1600 mg a day of SAMe had significantly better mood scores than women taking a placebo[1]. Ginkgo biloba may also help improve depression. When you improve depression and anxiety, you can greatly improve low libido.

Other good herbs include chastetree berry, licorice, and wild yam to balance hormones and get you back to feeling like yourself by correcting low hormones, out-of-balance hormones, changes in mood, and low libido. Also try motherwort and dandelion leaf and root. These can help by rebalancing the cycle and by detoxifying and clearing the liver.

For exhaustion, herbs such as suma and ginseng may help to build up depleted energy stores and return your body to normal.

The Thyroid Connection

Also consider that some women's thyroid glands can change after being pregnant, so if fatigue, depression, nervousness, constipation, intolerance of cold or heat, weight changes, muscle aches, changes in heart rate, menstrual changes, and/or irritability are particular issues, get your thyroid checked with a blood test and/or basal thermometer test. One out of twenty women will have a disorder of the immune system and develop antibodies against their own thyroid. These antibodies can damage the thyroid gland, causing it to malfunction—to function at too low or too high a level. This problem can last only briefly, or sometimes it can be permanent. Thyroid meds may be prescribed to get your energy back and deal with the accompanying depression and lack of libido.

Herbally, kelp, nori, dulse, and hijiki may be used to help normalize an under-active thyroid. A multivitamin/mineral formula, L-tyrosine, and selenium might help, as might zinc. If your thyroid is over-active, try the herbs lemon balm and bugleweed and perhaps vitamin A (don't use bugleweed if you are breast-feeding). Changes in the thyroid gland can cause lack of libido and depression, leading to lack of desire for sex, so it is important to have it checked to rule it out.

DID YOU KNOW?
ONE OUT OF TWENTY WOMEN WILL HAVE A DISORDER OF THE IMMUNE SYSTEM AND DEVELOP ANTIBODIES AGAINST THEIR OWN THYROID.

Except where noted, all the herbs mentioned in this chapter are safe to use while breast-feeding. Always check with a practitioner before taking nutrients/herbs if breast-feeding or consult our book Healthy Herbs: Your Everyday Guide to Medicinal Herbs and Their Use *(Fitzhenry &Whiteside 2006) or another authoritative herbal safety book.*

TREATMENT SUMMARY
Diet & Lifestyle
- Increase fruit, vegetables, whole grains, legumes, seeds, nuts, and unsaturated fats
- Eliminate caffeine, saturated fat, refined foods, and chemicals

Nutritional Supplements
- Multivitamin/mineral with a high dose of B vitamins
- Evening primrose oil: 1g twice a day

Herbs

- Red raspberry tea: infuse tea with 1-2 teaspoons and drink freely
- Use one, or a combination, of the following, relaxing nerviness:
  - Skullcap: 3g one to three times a day or 2-4ml tincture three times a day
  - Valerian: 1.5-2g as needed; 150-300mg extract standardized for 0.8% valeric acid once or twice a day; 1-3ml tincture three times a day
  - Chamomile: 3g (about a teaspoon) infused as a tea at least three times a day
  - Lemon balm: one teaspoon infused as a tea two to three times a day
  - Instead of chamomile tea or lemon balm tea alone, you can also use Rosemary Gladstar's Joy Tea

If depression is really a problem:

- Add one of:
  - St. John's wort: 300mg standardized extract three times a day
  - 5-HTTP: 50-100mg three times a day (if needed, you can go as high as 150mg four times a day)
  - SAMe: 400mg four times a day

If thyroid is the problem:

- Kelp and other seaweeds; 200mcg of selenium and 25mg of zinc if the thyroid is underactive
- Lemon balm (1.5-4.5g three times a day or one teaspoon infused as a tea two to three times a day) if the thyroid is overactive

ENDNOTE

1. Cerutti, R., *et al*. Psychological distress during puerperium. A novel therapeutic approach using S-adenosylmethionine. *Curr Ther Res* 1993; 53: 707–717.

Chapter Seven

MAKING MENOPAUSE EASY

So, it's that time and you have heard the horror stories for years. You watched your aunt, mother, and perhaps older sister go through this process, and now it's your turn, and you want there to be an easy, good way to go through menopause. Well, there is, and all those horror stories you have heard can be just that—stories. You can have a happy, easy, joyful, symptom-free menopause.

Menopause is a natural process that every woman will go through, and on the other side there is freedom, creativity, and more time for your change and growth!

So why is a chapter on menopause in a book on fertility and sexual health? Because for many women, menopause brings with it feelings of unattractiveness, low self-esteem, depression, anxiety, low libido, and physical symptoms such as vaginal dryness that make sex less likely to happen. But this chapter will show you how to avoid these issues so that you can stay sexually active your whole life.

Food, Culture, and Lifestyle

Women who eat a diet rich in whole foods, like lots of fresh fruits and vegetables, whole grains, legumes, and sea vegetables, and who avoid alcohol, caffeine, tobacco, and sugar have an easier time in menopause. This kind of diet provides better nutrition for the body and less build-up of toxins, and it simply leads to fewer menopausal symptoms such as hot flashes and anxiety and depression. It also helps to keep weight off, leading to more energy and fewer self-esteem issues.

Other help for menopausal symptoms, including hot flashes, comes from consuming a vegetarian diet that is high in fibre, antioxidants, and essential fatty acids, and low in unhealthy animal fats and trans fats. Try to eat more phytoestrogenic foods such as soy, fennel, celery, parsley, flax seeds, and other raw seeds and nuts. Have a soy burger, soy dog, or soy shake. Try delicious edamame or a stir-fry loaded with tofu. Add flax seeds to a soy smoothie or sprinkle them on salads and hot cereals. Eat tabouli with lots of parsley, or put parsley in fresh juices, and try fennel soup.

FOODS THAT FIGHT
HOT FLASHES
SOY
FENNEL
CELERY
PARSLEY
FLAX SEEDS

Women who exercise throughout life will also find their menopausal symptoms eased. Exercise helps to decrease blood cholesterol levels, decrease bone loss, improve ability to deal with stress, improve heart function, increase endurance, increase self-esteem, keep weight off, improve mood and cognitive and emotional stability, reduce blood pressure, relieve hot flashes, and increase oxygen and nutrient utilization of all tissues.

And women who take supplements and herbs to keep the body healthy also help to relieve their symptoms. Periodic internal cleansing of the body throughout life can aid during menopause. And don't forget to do something to relieve stress. All of these key factors play a huge role in relieving and preventing menopausal symptoms.

So much of the media focuses on the bad side effects of menopause, but a woman can go through menopause symptom-free. This time does not have to be spent in pain and discomfort, and it can be accomplished safely and without the scary side effects of the chemical hormones.

Yet, unfortunately, most women living in western culture, with all of its bad habits, often experience many unnecessary, uncomfortable, and disturbing changes when they go through menopause. Common symptoms such as hot flashes, night sweats, palpitations, and insomnia are experienced by most menopausal women in the west. Vaginal dryness and thinning is also common, as are depression, low self-esteem, loss of libido, and a number of other problems.

But, as we said, women do not need to suffer, nor do they need to go on dangerous chemical hormones to get relief. There is real help to be found. Natural health offers safe and effective relief. Diet and lifestyle and exercise are crucial to a healthy, symptom-free menopause. And for those who need a little extra help, there are a number of super herbs to provide it.

Super Menopause Plants
Plant Isoflavones
Isoflavones are plant nutrients found in soy that are weakly estrogenic, giving them an incredible ability: if your estrogen levels are low, as in menopause, they gently raise them, but if they are too high, as in breast cancer, they lower them by stealing receptor sites from your own more powerful estrogen. Studies have shown that soy isoflavones help not only with hot flashes, but also with vaginal dryness and thinning[1], breast cancer, and osteoporosis. They are also able to help with the psychological symptoms of menopause: soy isoflavones significantly improve feelings of depression, tiredness, and anger in menopausal women, as well as improving memory[2]. And they do this safely, unlike chemical estrogens.

Vaginal dryness and thinning can be an unpleasant and unwanted companion of menopause because there is no longer enough estrogen to produce the cells that line the vagina or to maintain moisture. This condition, known as atrophic vaginitis, can cause intercourse to become painful and unpleasant after menopause. When you get rid of the vaginal dryness and thinning, you are way more likely to be interested in sex—soy to the rescue! The ability of soy isoflavones to improve mood and energy can also aid libido.

A recent study has also found that red clover, another source of isoflavones, may have cardiovascular benefits for menopausal women.

Plant estrogens are easy to get in the diet. Try drinking soy milk, or try edamame, celery, flax seed, or fennel.

Menopause Superstar: Black Cohosh

This North American herb is the superstar for menopausal women. Once, black cohosh was believed to be what is called a phytoestrogenic herb: a herb that contains estrogen and can lower or raise your body's estrogen as needed, safely. But it is now known that it does not have those estrogenic properties. Yet, even without estrogen, this amazing herb continues to consistently outperform estrogen therapy in the treatment of menopause[3]. And, unlike the hormones, it does it safely and without side effects.

It is wonderfully effective against hot flashes, sweating, and heart palpitations. But, most importantly for the subject of this book, black cohosh is also able to help vaginal thinning and drying[4], problems that estrogen-replacement therapy has little effect on. And studies have also shown black cohosh to be extremely effective—better than hormones or valium—in treating the nervousness, irritability, depression, anxiety, and sleep disturbances that can come with menopause[5]. Again, you get rid of these physical and psychological symptoms, and you are way more likely to have good self-esteem, emotional stability, and improved libido.

Black cohosh might also be able to help with the osteoporosis associated with menopause[6].

Black cohosh shares with isoflavones the advantage over estrogen therapy of not stimulating breast tumours. Quite the opposite: black cohosh inhibits breast tumours and may prevent breast cancer[7], unlike chemical estrogens, which are believed to cause breast cancer.

Black cohosh also reduces or eliminates ringing in the ears, vertigo, sleep disturbances, joint pain, headache, and the profuse perspiration that can accompany menopause.

Another Menopause Superstar: Chastetree Berry

Perhaps the very best female tonic, chastetree berry is the great hormone balancer: it balances the ratio of estrogen to progesterone and so helps treat some of the underlying causes of many of the uncomfortable symptoms of menopause. It slightly favours progesterone over estrogen. Progesterone's role in relieving menopausal symptoms is often overlooked, yet progesterone is low in most menopausal women. This incredible herb helps with vaginal dryness, hot flashes, dizziness, and the depression of menopause. Along with black cohosh and soy, chastetree berry's ability to sooth vaginal dryness and depression makes it an important herb for menopause and sexuality.

Eastern Help: Dong Quai

This remarkable herb has a long history of use in China as a female remedy. Though not used alone for menopause, dong quai's role as a cardiovascular and hormonal tonic, as well as a nervine, makes it a useful herb in any menopause formula. It is often called the female ginseng and is used for every kind of female problem.

Dong quai normalizes hormones through its action on blood vessels, the liver, and the endocrine system. It is a strengthening and nourishing herb that is good for easing into menopause and for difficulties such as hot flashes that arise during menopause. Like the ginsengs, it has been used to give more energy and to improve libido.

Herbal Licorice

The use of licorice dates back many centuries, and it has been used for many different common female problems in both the east and the west. Licorice possesses estrogen-like activity that makes it a wonderful herb for treating menopause; however, it is also believed to raise progesterone levels—another important benefit for women in menopause—thus balancing the hormones. It is another great herb for getting rid of hot flashes and depression. And less depression and fewer hot flashes means better libido. It is a wonderful herb for building up depleted adrenal glands, too, making it great for stress and exhaustion and for improving mood.

Wild Yam

Wild yam is another herb that normalizes hormone production and regulates the balance of estrogen and progesterone. Since it is also a liver detoxifier, wild yam is especially useful when the liver as well as the reproductive system is behind the hormone imbalance.

Sage for Sweats

For menopausal women who suffer from hot flashes, sage is a must. This simple, well-known cooking herb is less known as an astringent that can dry up hot flashes, especially night sweats. It may be the best herb of all for drying menopausal sweats. Clinically, Linda has seen a simple sage tea work to get rid of hot flashes time and time again. Again, fewer hot flashes mean more energy and a better libido.

Cleaning the Liver

Why clean the liver during menopause? Because the liver is an important organ for the production, regulation, and detoxification of hormones. So herbs that work on the liver, such as dandelion, yellow dock, boldo, wild yam, and milk thistle, are excellent herbs for menopause. Get rid of toxins and your overall health and sense of well-being improve greatly.

Ginkgo Biloba

This herb is of great benefit to those who suffer from the cold hands and feet that are common in menopause and also the forgetfulness and lack of concentration. Ginkgo biloba increases circulation to the hands and feet, making these symptoms disappear. Ginkgo biloba may also help increase the libido that can fall off with menopause and it can aid in depression.

Depression, Anxiety, Loss of Libido, and Sleep Disturbances

Menopause can also bring a host of symptoms related to cognitive and emotional changes. Depression, anxiety, sleep disturbance, and loss of libido are common. St. John's wort, SAMe, 5-HTP, and passionflower can all help to reduce these symptoms. St. John's wort, SAMe, and 5-HTP can relieve the depression that can lead to feelings of low self-worth, inactivity, and loss of libido. They can also help with sleep disturbances and anxiety. Passionflower is great for reducing anxiety[8] and inducing sleep. Other anti-anxiety herbs include skullcap, hops, valerian, and lemon balm. They can also help with sleep. Supplementing the amino acid gamma-aminobutyric acid, or GABA, one of your body's calming neurotransmitters, can also help with anxiety and improve sleep. Some people suffering from depression, insomnia, and anxiety find the amino acid tyrosine beneficial. Other useful herbs for anxiety and sleeplessness are lady's slipper, catnip, verbena, and oats.

It is no surprise that the excellent antidepressant herb St. John's wort should help depression during menopause. A more surprising and welcome benefit is that it also reverses libido loss and boosts sexuality in menopausal women. Almost all women experience some loss of libido after menopause. But in an intriguing study, St. John's wort not only reduced the sweating, palpitations, and irritability of menopause—perhaps itself surprising—it also reversed lost libido. St. John's wort significantly reduced menopausal women's feelings of unattractiveness in an incredible 77 out of 82 cases. Women on St. John's wort were more likely to initiate sex. And, though at the beginning of the study many of the menopausal women said that they did not think sexuality was as important as they once had, a full 80% found that their sexuality was "substantially enhanced" when taking St. John's wort[9]. And that makes St. John's wort one of the great contributors to menopause and a long life of sexuality!

Another herb that seems able to help both the irritating psychological side of menopause and the loss of sexuality is that mysterious herb that just keeps coming up: maca. We have already seen that this Peruvian herb might help men suffering from erectile dysfunction, infertility, and loss of libido. We saw, too, in the folklore, potions, and aphrodisiacs chapter that both men and women have eaten it as a vegetable to increase fertility. And now a very small double-blind, placebo-controlled study has found that maca can not only significantly improve the anxiety and depression of menopause, but can also significantly decrease sexual dysfunction[10].

However, there is an important caveat. Although the maca, as we have already seen when it is used by men, did not affect hormones in this study, in two other studies[11], it did. In both of those studies, maca helped with the physical symptoms of menopause, but levels of female hormones were affected, including a concerning increase in the harmful estradiol form of estrogen. It seems that while maca does not itself contain plant estrogen or other hormones, it encourages their production by the body. Although this seems to greatly help with the symptoms of menopause, until the issue of increasing estradiol is clarified (as well as increasing the bad LDL in one study, too), we are suspending judgment on this herb for women. Black cohosh does the trick for symptoms both physical and psychological and St. John's wort bats clean up for self-image, libido, and sexuality, and both of them are entirely safe.

Herbs for Energy
Menopause can bring a loss of energy with it and, so, a loss of libido. Since the various forms of ginseng can help increase energy and help your body deal with both physical and emotional stress, they can help increase libido, as can ashwagandha, suma, Rhodiola, and eleuthero. These herbs can also reduce anxiety and bad feelings.

Vitamin and Mineral Help
All menopausal women should supplement their diets with a good-quality multivitamin and mineral complex. The multi will help to prevent deficiencies that can make things worse and can help to protect your heart and bones as well.

For hot flashes, try adding natural mixed tocopherol vitamin E and vitamin C with bioflavonoids. Vitamin E, both topically and internally, can also help with the pain and discomfort of intercourse that comes with the vaginal dryness and thinning of menopause.

Also add a B-complex for stress and heart health.

And don't forget bone-building nutrients such as calcium, magnesium, boron, manganese, vitamin D, the B-vitamins, vitamin K, and zinc. Keeping bones strong becomes crucial when you go through menopause, but it is important to start supporting your bones even before menopause. Good herbs for bone health include alfalfa, nettle, dandelion, and chamomile.

Menopause is only one phase of your life, and it can be easy and as good as any other phase. For many women, it can be a liberating time of great growth. Also, many women feel free, not having to worry about pregnancy and birth control any more. And, as you have now seen, it can also be a time of feeling good about yourself and of healthy, fulfilling, and discomfort-free sexuality.

Tuning in to your body and supplying it with what it needs to make the transition can make this important time of your life a happy, healthy, pain-free, symptom-free, productive one, full of vitality.

> **I know all about your woman's troubles there, Edith.... If you're gonna have the change of life, you gotta do it right now. I'm gonna give you just thirty seconds. Now c'mon and change.**
>
> **–Archie Bunker, "All In the Family"**
>
> **(Fortunately, attitudes have changed since then, and there are many natural treatment options)**

TREATMENT SUMMARY
Diet & Lifestyle
- Increase legumes, fruit, vegetables, whole grains, sea vegetables, fibre and essential fatty acids. Eat more vegetarian food.
- Decrease alcohol, caffeine, sugar, saturated fats, and trans fats
- Eat lots of soy or take supplements enough to provide 50-150mg of isoflavones
- Quit smoking
- Exercise

Nutritional Supplements

- Multivitamin/mineral with lots of B vitamins
- For hot flashes, add:
  - Mixed tocopherol vitamin E: 400-800IU
  - Vitamin C: 1,200mg
  - Bioflavonoids: 1,200mg

Herbs

- Black cohosh: two tablets standardized for 1mg 27-deoxyacteine twice a day
- Chastetree berry: 175-225mg extract standardized for 0.5% agnuside once or twice a day
- Licorice: 1-2g three times a day
- Sage: 1-3g three times a day or drink an infused tea three times a day
- If depression and/or loss of libido are a problem, add 300mg of standardized extract of St. John's wort to black cohosh

ENDNOTES

1. Messina, M., S. Barnes. The roles of soy products in reducing risk of cancer. *J Natl Cancer Inst* 1991; 83:541–46.

2. Casini, M. L., *et al*. Psychological assessment of the effects of treatment with phytoestrogens on postmenopausal women: a randomized, double-blind, crossover, placebo-controlled study. *Fertil Steril* 2006; 85:972–78.

3. Stolze, H. An alternative to treat menopausal complaints. *Gynecology* 1982; 1:14–16; Warnecke, G. Influencing menopausal symptoms with a phyto-therapeutic agent. Successful therapy with *Cimicifuga* mono-extract. *MedWelt* 1985; 36(2):871–74; Stoll, W. Phytopharmacon influences atrophic vaginal epithelium: double-blind study—*Cimicifuga* vs. estrogenic substances. *Therapeutikon* 1987; 1:23–31.

4. Stoll, W. Phytopharmacon influences atrophic vaginal epithelium: double-blind study—*Cimicifuga* vs. estrogenic substances. *Therapeutikon* 1987; 1:23–31; Duker, E., *et al*. Effects of extracts from *Cimicifuga racemosa* on gonadotropin release in menopausal women and ovariectomized rats. *Planta Med* 1991; 57:420–24.

5. Stolze, H. An alternative to treat menopausal complaints. *Gynecology* 1982; 1:14–16; Warnecke, G. Influencing menopausal symptoms with a phyto-therapeutic agent. Successful therapy with *Cimicifuga* mono-extract. *MedWelt* 1985; 36(2):871–74; Stoll, W. Phytopharmacon influences atrophic vaginal epithelium: double-blind study—*Cimicifuga* vs. estrogenic substances. *Therapeutikon* 1987; 1:23–31.

6. Wuttke, W., D. Seidlova-Wuttke, C. Gorkow. The *Cimicifuga* preparation BNO 1055 vs. conjugated estrogens in a double-blind placebo-controlled study: effects on menopause symptoms and bone markers. *Maturitas*. 2003:44 Suppl 1; 67–77.

7. Nesselhut, T., *et al*. Studies of the proliferative potency of phytodrugs with estrogen-like effect in breast cancer cells. *Arch Gyneco Obstet* 1993; 817–18; Hostanska, K., *et al*. *Cimicifuga racemosa* extract inhibits proliferation of es-

trogen receptor-positive and negative human breast carcinoma cell lines by induction of apoptosis. *Breast Cancer Res Treat*. March 2004; 84:151–60; Rebbeck, T. R. A retrospective case-control study of the use of hormone-related supplements and association with breast cancer. *Int J Cancer* 2007; 120:1523–28; Hirschberg, A. L., *et al.* An isopropanolic extract of black cohosh does not increase mammographic breast density or breast cell proliferation in postmenopausal women. *Menopause* 2007; 14:89–96.

8. Akhondzadeh, S., *et al.* Passionflower in the treatment of generalized anxiety: a pilot double-blind randomized controlled trial with oxazepam. *J Clin Pharm Ther* 2001; 26:363–67.

9. Grube, B., A. Walper, D. Wheately. St. John's Wort extract: efficacy for menopausal symptoms of psychological origin. *Adv Ther* 1999; 16:177–86.

10. Brooks, N. A., *et al.* Beneficial effects of *Lepidium meyanii* (maca) on psychological symptoms and measures of sexual dysfunction in postmenopausal women are not related to estrogen or androgen content. *Menopause: The Journal of the North American Menopause Society* 2008; 15:1157–62.

11. Meissner, H. O., *et al.* Hormone-balancing effect of pre-gelatinized organic maca (*Lepidium Peruvianum chacon*): (II) physiological and symptomatic responses of early-postmenopausal women to standard doses of maca in double-blind, randomized, placebo-controlled, multi-centre clinical study. *Int J Biomed Sci* 2006; 360–74; Meissner, H. O., *et al.* Hormone-balancing effect of pre-gelatinized organic maca (*Lepidium Peruvianum chacon*): (III) clinical responses of early-postmenopausal women to maca in double-blind, randomized, placebo-controlled, crossover configuration, outpatient study. *Int J Biomed Sci* 2006; 2:375–94.

Chapter Eight

PREVENTING AND TREATING URINARY TRACT INFECTIONS

Remember the movie *The Green Mile*? It starts with the main character, played by Tom Hanks, in great pain, needing to pee and unable to perform this key function. It isn't until a miracle happens that he returns to his old self again. He goes to the washroom, having been cured by a miracle, and in every way, returns to his healthy self. If you can't pee or if it hurts to pee or if you are peeing all the time, it is pretty hard to have sex or really to function in any normal way. This is why this chapter is in the book: because most people will have this problem at some point in their lives, often more than once, and it can interfere with all of life's normal processes.

More and more, people are getting not only one, but repeated urinary tract infections. Why? There are many reasons, but one of the most common is that the antibiotics that are used to treat urinary tract infections not only wipe out the bad bacteria, they also wipe out the good ones that protect against urinary tract infections. This often will cause the bacterial infection to repeat again and again. Also, bacteria are often resistant to antibiotics. So clearly, this very real problem needs a better way of being treated.

What's This Chapter Doing Here?

This chapter is in this book because urinary tract infections are so epidemic and can be so destructive that they can interfere with sex and even cause difficulties in getting pregnant. I frequently see women in my clinic who are trying to get pregnant, or even just to have sex, and cannot because of severe pain and burning from repeated urinary tract infections that have not been cured by antibiotics. Also, infections can cause scar tissue in both the male and female reproductive tract, low sperm count and motility in men, and hormonal imbalances that can cause infertility in both men and women. And sex itself can bring on infections: 60% of all cases of recurrent cystitis are caused by intercourse, and your chances of getting cystitis are way higher within the two days following intercourse.

There is a Monty Python skit about men running a race—a race for men with urinary incontinence. The gun goes off and the men start to run, and every few seconds one of them pulls off to the side of the track to go the washroom, off camera, of course. An extreme case, perhaps. But if the male organ is constantly doing one thing, it can't perform its other function at the same time.

So what does a urinary tract infection feel like? You constantly feel that you need to go to the washroom. And when you do go, it burns, comes out in spurts and, no matter how many times you empty your bladder, it still feels full. You can also feel tired and fluey.

It is one of the most common problems to affect women, often at least once a year. According to naturopathic doctors Michael Murray and Joseph Pizzorno, "10-20% percent of all woman have urinary tract discomfort at least once a year; 37.5% of woman with no history of urinary tract infections will have one within 10 years; and 2-4% of apparently healthy women have elevated levels of bacteria in their urine, indicative of an unrecognized urinary tract infection"[1]. Fifty-five per cent of women with recurrent bladder infections will eventually have involvement of the kidneys, which, for some, can mean scarring and even kidney failure. But it is not a woman's problem alone. Urinary tract infection can be a cause of male infertility. Urinary tract infections are less common in men, though, and often indicate an anatomical abnormality or a prostate infection that is causing the infertility.

The Many Causes of Urinary Tract Infections

There are many possible causes of urinary tract infections: bacteria enter-
ing the urinary tract through the bloodstream, bacteria ascending from the
urethra from faecal contamination or vaginal secretions, or, for men, prostate
problems. Those who suffer from pooling of the urine caused by obstructions
or anatomical problems are also at risk, as are those whose immune systems
are down. Those with candida are also at risk. And just having sex can pose a
risk from contamination. Stress and poor diet can also bring on the problem.

The diagnosis of urinary tract infections can also be difficult, since people
suffering from symptoms often do not have significant amounts of bacteria
in their urine. For example, 40% of women who have typical symptoms of
urinary tract infections do not have a significant amount of bacteria in their
urine[2].

Diagnosis of a urinary tract infection is usually made by a combination of
urinalysis and symptoms. Typical symptoms include lower back pain, fever,
chills, burning upon urination, urgency of urination, painful urination, odour
of the urine, cloudy urine, frequent urination, blood in the urine, nausea,
and frequent night-time urination. Although some may have few if any symptoms, they could still be infected.

While conventional medicine uses antibiotics to treat urinary tract infections, antibiotics may actually promote recurrent infections by promoting
the growth of antibiotic-resistant strains of bacteria[3]. People who suffer from
recurrent urinary tract infections often have bacteria that are resistant to
many antibiotics[4], which forces conventional doctors to prescribe more powerful and dangerous antibiotics that can cause adverse reactions. Antibiotics
disturb the friendly flora in the vagina, and since the flora in the vagina protect the bladder from harmful bacteria, this action of antibiotics can increase
the risk of further infections and of yeast infections. For most infections, the
natural approach is the best route to ensure not only that the infection goes
away, but that it does not come back.

For many people with recurrent bladder infections, the immune system is involved, so it is important to restore proper immune function. The diet should

consist of fresh whole foods and you should avoid sugar, caffeine, alcohol, soft drinks, chemicals in food, and refined carbohydrates, since these can all weaken the immune system and encourage the growth of bacteria. Also avoid food allergens, since they too can cause recurrent bladder irritations. I have found that those sensitive to gluten should avoid it, especially during an infection, as it can cause a dampness in the system and weaken it, leading to further infections. For some, avoiding dairy helps.

Sometimes just the switch to a healthier diet can strengthen the immune system, but often more immune help is needed.

Natural Help for Urinary Tract Infections

Perhaps the best herb for enhancing immunity is Echinacea. All kinds of studies have shown that Echinacea has several powerful effects on the immune system[5]. Echinacea is useful for urinary tract infections, especially when combined with other herbs.

HERBS THAT SUPPORT
THE IMMUNE SYSTEM
LICORICE
EUROPEAN MISTLETOE
GINSENG
GOLDENSEAL
BONESET
GARLIC
ASTRAGALUS
LIGUSTRUM,

If it is specifically the thymus gland, the key gland of the immune system, that is behind the immune weakness, licorice and European mistletoe can be of use, according to Michael Murray, N.D. There are many other helpful herbs and nutrients that can help to support the immune system, such as ginseng, goldenseal, boneset, garlic, astragalus, ligustrum, vitamin C, B6, beta-carotene, and zinc. It is also a good idea to ensure that your immune system is getting all the crucial nutrients it needs to prevent infections from recurring by taking a high-quality multivitamin/mineral every day.

Cranberry Juice

One of the best things you can do to treat a urinary tract infection is to drink lots of liquids. And the best liquid for urinary tract infections is unsweetened cranberry juice. Cranberry juice and cranberry-juice supplements have been used to treat urinary tract infections for years. They have been shown in studies to be very effective. In one study, sixteen ounces of cranberry juice per day was consumed by people with urinary tract infections. Seventy-three per cent of patients with active urinary tract infections showed improvement. And when patients stopped consuming cranberry juice, 61% of them experienced a recurrence of bladder infections[6]. It is now known that cranberry juice does not work on infections by acidifying the urine as was once believed. Cranberry juice works in a far more interesting way—it actually prevents the bacteria from adhering to the walls of the urinary tract, so it literally can't stick around and infect the body[7]. Dr. Edwin Kass of Harvard says that, "Cranberry juice can eliminate bacteria even in those whose bladder infections have been resistant to previous antibiotic therapy"[8]. Blueberry[9], raspberry, strawberry, and currant juice also work. Aloe juice can also help.

As we have already seen, urinary tract infections can not only cause problems with fertility and for sexual intercourse, but sexual intercourse can cause urinary tract infections. Infections are far more common after sex. So, can cranberry juice prevent post-sex urinary tract infections? Yup. Researchers gave either 500 mg of cranberry powder or a placebo to 111 women with recurrent lower urinary tract infections who had intercourse more than once every two weeks. The pills were given six hours after intercourse. While 43.2% of the women in the placebo group had a recurrent lower urinary tract infection, a remarkably few 10.8% of the women in the cranberry group did[10]. So, try cranberries after sex. Try them fresh, too.

It is also a good idea to wipe the vaginal area, from front to back, with a diluted solution of goldenseal powder mixed with spring water before and after sex. Men who are susceptible to infections can wipe the penis with the solution, too.

Uva Ursi

Uva ursi is one of the most commonly used herbs to treat urinary tract infections. It is also one of the very best. It is effective against *E. coli*, the bacteria that causes about 90% of all urinary tract infections, and other urinary-tract-infection-causing bacteria. Traditionally, it has been used to treat bladder and kidney infections, kidney stones, and edema. Uva ursi does it all. It is a diuretic, urinary antiseptic and astringent that is useful for urinary tract infections and for blood in the urine. Clinically, I have found uva ursi to be one of the most important herbs for most common infections of the urinary tract and often suggest people use it on and off for a while to wipe out the infection and to prevent it from coming back. It is also used for prostate infections that can cause infertility in men. Uva ursi should not be used if you may be pregnant.

Garlic

Garlic is effective against several of the bacteria associated with urinary tract infections, including E. coli, Proteus spp., Klebsiella pneumonia, and Staphylococus spp.[11]. It is a good idea to consume plenty of fresh garlic, too. This herb has proven itself to be especially effective against stubborn infections or lingering infections, and it strengthens the immune system, so it helps in this way, too.

Goldenseal

Goldenseal has a long history of use in the treatment of all infections, including urinary tract infections, for which it is a powerful herb. Studies have shown it to be effective against E. coli, Proteus spp., Klebsiella spp., Staphylococcus spp., Enterobacter aerogenes, and Pseudomonas spp[12]. As well as the direct antibiotic properties of goldenseal, it has been shown to prevent the adhesion of the bacteria[13]. It also improves immunity and works on vaginal and prostrate infections, which can be related. Goldenseal should not be used if you may be pregnant.

Buchu

Buchu has been used for centuries in South Africa for urinary, kidney, and prostate problems. It is used to relieve inflammation of the kidneys, cramps in the bladder, and to sooth and strengthen the urinary organs. Herbalist Michael Tierra calls it one of the best diuretics known and recommends it for both acute and chronic urinary tract problems. For men's infections, I often combine it with corn silk. Buchu is probably safe during pregnancy, though herbs sometimes confused with or substituted for buchu are not. So be careful, or just use one of the many other herbs.

Cleavers

Cleavers is a very good diuretic that is useful for all urinary problems. Old-time herbalists used this herb for scalding urine, dropsy, irritation at the neck of the bladder, and stones in the bladder.

Corn silk

Corn silk is a demulcent diuretic that sooths the urinary tract. Its antiseptic powers are useful for cleansing the urinary tract, making it useful for treating urinary tract infections.

You can try Herbalist Michael Tierra's formula:
1 part of each of buchu, uva ursi, parsley root, cleavers, juniper berries, marshmallow root, and ¼ part ginger root. Combine the herbs and simmer one ounce of herbs in one pint of water for twenty minutes. Take half a cup of the tea four times per day after meals and before going to bed. He calls this formula a bladder/kidney tonic, good for the whole genito-urinary tract and a good diuretic.

Paul Pitchford, author of *Healing with Whole Foods*, suggests using spirulina, marshmallow herb, rehmannia root, asparagus root, and aloe vera gel to strengthen the kidneys and keep them strong. Eleuthero, formerly known as Siberian ginseng, can also help to strengthen the system and keep the immune system strong.

There are many other useful herbs for the urinary tract, including juniper berries, parsley, pau d'arco, saw palmetto, marshmallow, goldenrod, plantain, wild carrot, gravel root (especially for stones of the kidney), and white poplar bark (useful for urinary weakness, especially in the elderly, or for anyone who has weak kidneys or incontinence). It is not necessary to use all of them, but rather choose one or a few and combine them either to strengthen the urinary tract, treat infections or stones, or to clean the urinary system.

ENDEAVOUR TO ELIMINATE A URINARY TRACT INFECTION BEFORE TRYING TO BECOME PREGNANT

Endeavour to eliminate the infection before trying to become pregnant. If you are, or may be pregnant, be sure to confirm that the herb you have chosen is safe during pregnancy. Consult our book, *Healthy Herbs: Your Everyday Guide to Medicinal Herbs and Their Use* (Fitzhenry & Whiteside 2006) or another authoritative book on herbal safety and contraindications.

To keep the immune system functioning at its peak and to keep infections from coming back, acidophilus and bifidus are very important. People with low friendly flora from overuse of antibiotics are especially at risk for recurrent urinary tract infections. Those with candida should definitely take probiotics and also treat for candida (see candida chapter). Use 20 billion live cells a day during an infection and for at least two weeks after that. Vaginal inserts of probiotics can also help, since both systems are closely connected.

If you have a urinary tract infection, it is a good idea to help support the immune system by taking about 5 g of buffered vitamin C mixed with bioflavonoids (1 g per day) and zinc, 30 to 50 mg per day, until it is cleared up.

If an infection is present, wear only underwear made from cotton; use plain unbleached toilet paper; keep the area clean; for women, avoid tampons; and be sure to empty the bladder as soon as the urge to do so is present.

Drink plenty of water: increasing urine flow to keep the system flushed out is important.

Also make use of sitz baths to help relieve the irritation and fight the infection. Men with low sperm count/motility should probably not use the sitz baths. You can also use acupuncture to help get rid of an infection and to strengthen the system.

TREATMENT SUMMARY
Diet & Lifestyle
- Drink lots of water
- Eat lots of garlic
- Avoid sugar, caffeine, alcohol, soft drinks, refined carbohydrates, and food allergens

Nutritional Supplements
- Vitamin C (buffered): 5g a day

- Bioflavonoids: 1g a day
- Zinc: 30-50mg a day
- Probiotics: 20 billion live cells a day

Herbs

- Cranberry juice (unsweetened): 16 ounces a day; 10-16 400-500mg pills a day; or 400mg concentrated extract two to three times a day
- Echinacea: 2-5ml of the tincture three times a day or thirty drops every two hours
- If you are pregnant and want to add something to the cranberry and Echinacea, try garlic and/or corn silk
- Choose one, or a combination, of the following, if you are not pregnant:
  - Uva ursi: 10-12g a day or 250-500mg solid extract standardized for 10% arbutin
  - Goldenseal: 1-2g three times a day or 250-500mg standardized for 8-12% alkaloids three times a day

ENDNOTES

1. Pizzorno, J. E., M. T. Murray, eds. Textbook of Natural Medicine, 2nd ed. London, UK: Churchill Livingstone, 1999, p.1183.

2. Reilly, B. M. Practical Strategies in Outpatient Medicine. Philadelphia, PA: W.B. Saunders, 1984, p. 277. Cited in Pizzorno, J. E., M. T. Murray, eds. Textbook of Natural Medicine, 2nd ed. London, UK: Churchill Livingstone, 1999, p.1184.

3. Balch, J. F., P. A. Balch. *Prescription for Nutritional Healing*. Garden City Park, NY: Avery, 1997, p.159.

4. Schmidt, M. A., L. H. Smith, K. W. Sehnert. *Beyond Antibiotics: 50 (or so) Ways to Boost Immunity and Avoid Antibiotics*. Berkeley, CA: North Atlantic Books, 1994, p.227.

5. Woolven, L., T. Snider. *Healthy Herbs:Your Everyday Guide to Medicinal Herbs and Their Use*. Markham, ON: Fitzhenry & Whiteside, 2006, pp.57–60.

6. Prodromos, P. N., C. A. Brusch, G. C. Ceresia. Cranberry juice in the treatment of urinary tract infections. *Southwest Med* 1968; 47:17.

7. Sobota, A. E. Inhibition of bacteria adherence by cranberry juice: potential use for the treatment of urinary tract infections. *J Urol* 1984; 131:1013–16; Ofek, I., *et al*. Anti-escherichia coli adhesion activity of cranberry and blueberry juices. *N Engl J Med* 1991; 324:1599.

8. Schmidt, M. A., L. H. Smith, K. W. Sehnert. *Beyond Antibiotics: 50 (or so) Ways to Boost Immunity and Avoid Antibiotics*. Berkeley, CA: North Atlantic Books, 1994, p. 27.

9. Ofek, I., *et al*. Anti-escherichia coli adhesion activity of cranberry and blueberry juices. *N Engl J Med* 1991; 324:1599.

10. Bohbot, J.-M. Results of a randomized, double-blind study on the prevention of recurrent cystitis with GynDelta®. *Gynaecologist's Obstetrician's*

11. Sharma, V. D., *et al.* Antibacterial property of *Allium sativum* Linn. In vivo & in vitro studies. *Ind J Exp Biol* 1977; 15:466–68; Adetumbi, M. A., B. H. Lau. *Allium sativum* (garlic)—a natural antibiotic. *Med Hypothesis* 1983; 12:227–37; Elnima, E. I., *et al.* The antimicrobial activity of garlic and onion extracts. *Pharmazie* 1983; 38:747–48.

12. Johnson, C. C., G. Johnson, C. F. Poe. Toxicity of alkaloids to certain bacteria. *Acta Pharmacol Toxicol* 1952; 8:71–78; Amin, A. H., T. V. Subbaiah, K. M. Abbasi. Berberine sulfate: Antimicrobial activity, bioassay, and mode of action. *Can J Microbiol* 1969; 15:1067–76.

13. Sun, D. X., S. N. Abraham, E. H. Beachey. Influence of berberine sulfate on synthesis and expression of pap fimbrial adhesion in uropathogenic *Escherichia coli. Antimicrob Agents Chemother* 1988; 32:1274–77; Sun, D., H. S. Courtney, E. H. Beachey. Berberine sulfate blocks adherence of Streptococcus pyogenes to epithelial cells, fibronectin, and headecane. *Antimicrobial Agents Chemother* 1988; 32:1370–74.

Chapter Nine

CANDIDA

What is candida? It is an overgrowth of yeast that causes a whole host of symptoms—yeast infections, jock itch, rashes, tiredness, confusion, weakness, low immune function, headaches, poor digestion, malabsorption, allergies, anxiety, sensitivities to chemicals, perfumes, rubber and more, and gynecological problems, among other problems. Why is it in a book on sexual health and fertility? Because some have linked it with female problems that can make fertility more difficult, such as endometriosis, fibroids, fibrocystic breast disease, ovarian cysts, and, of course, vaginal pain, irritation, and lack of desire for sex. It may be linked to low sperm counts and motility issues in men, too. And it is linked to depression, stress, and anxiety, which can make getting pregnant difficult. Stress is the number-one cause of cases of infertility of unknown origin.

The Causes of Candida: Drugs and Diet
What causes candida? The overuse of antibiotics is the most important factor in its development[1]. Antibiotics not only kill the disease-causing bacteria, but the beneficial ones as well. By suppressing beneficial intestinal bacteria, antibiotics promote yeast overgrowth and suppress the immune system. Having

a suppressed immune system means you are more likely to develop candida and bacterial infections. Then they put you on more antibiotics, leading to more candida. It can be a vicious cycle for many people.

And there are other drugs, for instance, corticosteroids, oral contraceptives, and ulcer medicines that cause candida. One study found that ulcer medications such as Zantac and Tagamet actually cause candida overgrowth in the stomach[2]. These medicines are designed to suppress hydrochloric acid, showing how important hydrochloric acid is in preventing candida. To correct low stomach acid, try supplementing hydrochloric acid or taking herbal bitters. Bitters help to promote hydrochloric acid in the stomach, helping to prevent candida. You can also try apple cider vinegar for this problem. Gentian is one of our favourite herbs for bringing up low stomach acid and toning the whole digestive system.

FOODS THAT PROMOTE YEAST OVERGROWTH

SIMPLE CARBOHYDRATES
REFINED SUGARS
FRUIT JUICES
HONEY
MAPLE SYRUP
YEAST
FOODS WITH MOULD
ALCOHOL
DRIED FRUIT
MELONS
MILK & MILK PRODUCTS

Candida feeds mainly on sugar, so the sugar- and refined-carbohydrate-laden diet that many of us consider normal is another important cause of candida.

Curing Candida
Diet to the Rescue

So, as you can see, stomach acid is important in treating and preventing candida. Also, diet is key. A diet that avoids simple carbohydrates, refined sugars, fruit juices, honey, maple syrup, yeast, foods with mould (like peanuts), alcohol, dried fruit, melons, and milk and milk products—since they contain lactose, or milk sugar—works well to fight candida and to prevent it. Getting rid of sugar is the most crucial step in getting rid of candida[3]. The good news is that these dietary changes will not only help you to fight candida, but will also help you to become pregnant; remember that eating complex carbs but avoiding refined carbs was one of the crucial moves for increasing female fertility (see female infertility chapter). Also limit your intake of high-carbohydrate foods like potatoes and corn. Go ahead and eat all the other vegetables, legumes, and whole non-glutinous grains you want. Be careful of gluten, though; it can aggravate the colon and weaken the immune system, and, for many people, it is an allergen. So try some of the more exotic and delicious grains like quinoa, amaranth, teff, buckwheat, millet, and brown rice. You can even enjoy some fruit, such as apples, pears, and berries, but limit it to two to three cups a day. And, of course, avoid all known or suspected food allergens, since they can weaken the immune system, allowing candida to overgrow.

The Liver Connection

The liver doesn't seem to function well in people with candida, causing such problems as sensitivities to chemicals and, often, PMS and skin problems, since the liver can't do its job of filtering the blood properly. A damaged liver allows candida overgrowth, and while your program is successfully killing off the candida, the dying candida produce toxins that need a strong liver to filter them out. So it is really important to support the liver as part of your candida program. Use liver-supporting herbs such as black radish, turmeric, milk thistle, gentian or other bitters, artichokes, Oregon grape root, goldenseal, and dandelion root. Jerusalem artichokes are high in FOS (fructo-oligosac-charides), another key ingredient in fighting off candida.

Candida-Killing Supplements

Some of the most common supplements used in fighting candida are caprylic acid, bentonite, and acidophilus. Acidophilus, along with several other strains of probiotics, is crucial. Acidophilus replenishes the friendly flora in the gut, where they help to kill the candida and improve the digestion and absorption of nutrients, as well as helping to correct a weakened immune system and any nutritional deficiencies that can cause candida. Be sure to get a very high-quality probiotic supplement. And look for one that has FOS added. Studies show that FOS increases the friendly bacteria bifidobacteria and lactobacilli, while reducing detrimental bacteria[4]. It also improves liver function and improves the elimination of toxic compounds, which is crucial in the treatment of candida. Caprylic acid helps to kill the overgrowth[5], and bentonite clay helps to remove toxins from the colon.

Another good choice in fighting candida is grapefruit-seed extract; it can be used safely for months at a time. It is useful for getting rid of the candida yeast that has spread throughout the body. Michael Rosenbaum, M.D., and Murray Susser, M.D., authors of *Solving the Puzzle of Chronic Fatigue Syndrome*, say grapefruit-seed extract has a powerful action on candida. Linda has seen it work wonders on candida in her clinic, and it is often the first thing she will suggest.

One of the most effective herbs against candida is goldenseal. Goldenseal is high in berberine, which is effective against candida and many bacterial infections, including urinary tract infections. So if you are susceptible to urinary tract infections and candida, this one herb can do both jobs, and help you to avoid antibiotics that can weaken the system and lead to candida. Goldenseal is also excellent in stopping the diarrhoea that can come with candida, and it will increase immune function, helping to destroy viruses, yeast, and bacteria. It normalizes intestinal flora, helps with digestive problems, and stimulates the immune system. Some claim that goldenseal works better than any other therapy in killing off the candida. Barberry and Oregon grape root have similar properties.

Also try pau d'arco, oregano oil, garlic, and cinnamon—all excellent candida fighters. Pau d'arco has been used traditionally in South America for years to improve the immune system, and it is powerful against candida[6]. Garlic is one of the best and easiest natural foods to take to kill off candida[7], and you can also use it as a supplement. Oregano oil is hugely popular now, and it kills off the candida extremely effectively[8] while it also strengthens the immune system. Cinnamon is another great and easy-to-use candida fighter, as a food or as a herbal supplement.

Among other herbs and spices that are discussed as effective antifungal agents and candida fighters are German chamomile, uva ursi, aloe vera, ginger, rosemary, thyme balm (not *time bomb*, although they each may be a time bomb for candida), licorice, fennel, hyssop, calendula, marjoram, oregano, and tea tree oil.

Or try a little known herb called mathake, or tropical almond. It is commonly used in the South Pacific and is supposed to be one of the most effective antifungal agents there is. William Crook suggests this herb in his book,

The Yeast Connection and the Woman, and Rosenbaum and Susser mention it in *Solving the Puzzle of Chronic Fatigue Syndrome*.

Also be sure to have plenty of fibre in your diet to ensure clean bowels. Undigested material that is left to sit in the colon can ferment, leading to an overgrowth of yeast. You might want to add flax seeds, pectin, or psyllium to your diet to keep the bowels clean. Fibre also positively affects the balance of good and bad bacteria. Eat lots of brown rice for a good non-allergic source of fibre.

While you are killing off the yeast, be sure to supplement with vitamins and minerals to help correct any nutritional deficiencies that may have weakened your immune system, allowing candida to take over your body. At the very least, take a high-potency multivitamin and mineral formula.

Immune Connection

To strengthen your immune system and to prevent the reoccurrence of vulvo-vaginal candida, try adding Echinacea purpurea to your candida regime[9]. You can also try using other immune-enhancing herbs, such as astragalus, dong quai, licorice, ginseng, and wild indigo to keep your immune system strong and to prevent candida.

Drugs and Candida

As for the traditional drugs that are used against candida, Dr. Virender Sodhi says the most popularly used drug, nystatin, does not get rid of candida, even after it has been in use for one year, but only causes it to mutate into another species of yeast. And he says that nystatin lingers in the intestine and can kill other helpful organisms[10].

The good news is that garlic, an extremely powerful antibacterial and antifungal agent, has been shown to be more effective than nystatin in treating candida[11]. Diluted garlic can even be applied to tampons and used as a vaginal insert to get rid of vaginitis. Or try diluted gentian violet on tampons or as a wash and douche. Grapefruit-seed extract, diluted, also works well vaginally, as does diluted boric acid.

For topical relief of irritation and burning for either partner, try aloe vera juice or balm, calendula cream, licorice, or slippery elm powder made into a poultice. This will also make sex less painful and irritating. If you have candida, most likely your partner does too, so treat both to get rid of the problem.

If your candida is linked to endometriosis, fibroids, or cysts that are causing you problems with fertility, see Linda's book, *Smart Woman's Guide to PMS and Pain-free Periods* for comprehensive, easy-to-follow treatments for those problems.

TREATMENT SUMMARY
Diet & Lifestyle
- Avoid sugar, simple carbohydrates, fruit juice, honey, maple syrup, yeast, alcohol, dried fruit, peanuts, cashews, dairy, tropical fruits, melons, oranges, and grapes.
- You can include apples, pears, berries, peaches, plums, seeds, and nuts
- Freely eat complex carbohydrates, vegetables, legumes, non-glutenous grains (quinoa, amaranth, buckwheat, millet, brown rice) and plenty of fibre

Nutritional Supplements
- Probiotics: 20 billion live cells a day
- FOS: 2,000-3,000mg a day
- High potency multivitamin/mineral

Herbs
- Milk thistle standardized for 70-80% silymarin: 140mg of silymarin two to three times a day (or other liver-supporting herb)
- Take one, or a combination, of:
  - Grapefruit seed extract: 5-15 drops three times a day
  - Goldenseal: 1-2g three times a day or 250-500mg standardized for 8-12% alkaloids three times a day (do not use goldenseal if you are pregnant)
  - Garlic: 300mg three times a day
  - Pau d'arco: 900mg three times a day or 3-6 cups of a decoction

- Oregano oil: 0.2-0.4ml in enteric-coated capsules twice a day

ENDNOTES

1. Caruso, L. J. Vaginal moniliasis after tetracycline therapy. *Am J Obstet Gynecol* 1964; 90:374; Reid, G., A. W. Bruce, R. L. Cook. Effect on urogenital flora of antibiotic therapy of urinary tract infection. *Scand J Infect Dis* 1990; 22:43–47; Nord, C. E, C. Edlund. Impact of antimicrobial agents on human intestinal microflora. *J Chemother* 1990; 2:218–237.

2. Buero, M., *et al.* Candida overgrowth in gastric juice of peptic ulcer subjects on short- and long-term treatment with H2-receptor antagonists. *Digestion* 1983; 28:158–63.

3. Horowitz. B. J., S. Edelstein, L. Lippman. Sugar chromatography studies in recurrent Candida vulvovaginitis. *J Reprod Med* 1984; 29:441–43.

4. Murray, M. T. *Chronic Candidiasis: The Yeast Syndrome.* Rocklin, CA: Prima Publishing, 1997, p. 120.

5. Keeney, E. L. Sodium caprylate: a new and effective treatment of moniliasis of the skin and mucous membrane. *Bull Johns Hopkins Hosp* 1946; 78:333–9; Neuhauser, I., E. L. Gustus. Successful treatment of intestinal moniliasis with fatty acid resin complex. *Arch Intern Med* 1954; 93:53–60.

6. Gershon, H., L. Shanks. Fungitoxicity of 1,4-naphthoquinones to Candida albicans and trichophyton mentagrphytes. *Can J Microbiol* 1975; 21:1317–21; De Lima, O. G., *et al. Rev Inst Antibiot (Recife)* 1971; 11:21–26; Oswald, E. H. *Br J Phytother* 1993/1994; 3:112–27.

7. Arora, D. S., J. Kaur. Anti-microbial activity of spices. *Int J Antimicrob Agents* 1999; 12:257–62.

8. Stiles, J. C. The inhibition of Candida albicans by oregano. *J Applied Nutr* 1995; 47:96–102.

9. Coeugniet, E., R. Kuhnast. Recurrent candidiases: Adjuvant immu-

notherapy with different formulations of Echinacin. *Therapiewoche* 1986; 36:3352–58.

10. The Burton Goldberg Group. *Alternative Medicine: The Definitive Guide.* Fife, WA: Future Medicine Publishing, 1995, p.591.

11. Arora, D. S., J. Kaur. Anti-microbial activity of spices. *Int J Antimicrob Agents* 1999; 12:257–62.

Chapter Ten

BENIGN PROSTATIC HYPERPLASIA: ENLARGED PROSTATE

You saw Grandpa get up several times a night to go to the washroom, and then, as he got older, your dad. You are hoping to avoid the same thing.

Either gradually or suddenly, most men find that they wake up at night to urinate and that they are going more frequently throughout the day. It may even be difficult to fully empty the bladder. If this sounds like you, you just may have benign prostatic hyperplasia.

If you are between the ages of forty and fifty-nine and are male, you have a 60% chance of developing an enlarged prostate, a condition known as benign prostatic hyperplasia (BPH). By the time you are in your eighth decade, your chances of developing BPH go up to over 90%.

The prostate is the gland that surrounds the urethra, the exit by which the urine leaves the bladder. When it is enlarged due to an increased concentration of a potent form of testosterone known as dihydrotestosterone, it can cause an increase in many symptoms, including the frequent need to urinate, night-time awakening to urinate, reduced flow of urine, urgency, pain, or difficulty upon urinating, inability to fully empty the bladder, and obstruction of the bladder outlet, which can lead to retention of urine in the blood, kidney infections, and weakness.

BPH can interfere with sex because of pain and discomfort and because of exhaustion from waking up at night to urinate. And since one organ performs double duty, you don't want it always to be doing that one! BPH can also cause hormonal changes that may alter both the desire for and the ability to have sex, so this is why this chapter is included in the book. A healthy prostate is an important, but often overlooked, part of a healthy reproductive system. Prostate problems can be involved in both erectile dysfunction and infertility. It is especially crucial for fertility because the fluid secreted by the prostate gland is essential for optimal sperm motility.

Zinc and the Right Fats

Many believe diet plays an important role in the treatment and prevention of BPH. Studies have shown that a diet high in zinc can reduce the size of the prostate[1]. It is believed that zinc, which is found in a healthy prostate at levels higher than anywhere else in the body, helps to metabolize male hormones within the prostate and to prevent the production of dihydrotestosterone, allowing the prostate to return to its normal size. Supplementation of zinc for BPH should be 50 mg a day, and its benefit can be increased if you take vitamin B6. You should also add 2 to 3 mg of copper a day when supplementing with this amount of zinc long-term. Zinc just may help you do two things at once, since we have already seen how crucial it is for male fertility.

> **DID YOU KNOW?**
> A DIET THAT INCLUDES UP TO HALF A CUP A DAY OF PUMPKIN SEEDS CAN HELP TO REDUCE PROSTATE ENLARGEMENT.

Other crucial nutrients important in the treatment of BPH include essential fatty acids like the kind found in pumpkin seeds. A diet that includes up to half a cup a day of pumpkin seeds can help to reduce prostate enlargement, since the seeds are not only high in essential fatty acids but are also high in zinc. Pumpkin seeds also contain chemicals that may prevent the formation of dihydrotestosterone. Flax-seed oil, safflower oil, evening primrose oil, hemp oil, and soy oil are all good sources of essential fatty acids. Essential fatty acids are believed to help by being precursors to prostaglandins, which can help to stop testosterone from causing increased growth of the prostate[2].

Herbs

Saw Palmetto: Superstar for BPH

The most exciting herb for treating BPH is saw palmetto. In fact, the most exciting anything for treating BPH is saw palmetto. Traditionally, saw palmetto has been used by the First Nations people of North America as a treatment for various urinary troubles. The extract made from the berries of the saw palmetto palm tree has been found to reduce symptoms associated with BPH better than the commonly used drugs finasteride (Proscar) and tamsulosin (Flomax).

Saw palmetto is not only more effective than the drugs, but safer. And for our purposes, this enhanced safety is crucial, because a common side effect of BPH drugs is none other than erectile dysfunction. Several head-to-head studies have shown saw palmetto berry extract does the job as well or better, with a hugely reduced risk of this unwelcome side effect[3].

Typically, a dosage of 320 mg a day for at least three months makes the symptoms of BPH go away for up to 90% of sufferers. Numerous studies involving patients suffering from BPH have shown excellent results using saw palmetto extract[4]. To receive the full benefit of saw palmetto, it should be standardized to contain 85% to 95% fatty acids and sterols.

You might also remember from the chapter on folklore, potions, and aphrodisiacs that saw palmetto has also shown up as an aphrodisiac, so, who knows?

Pygeum

Another herb that is especially good for many men with BPH is pygeum, from the bark of a tropical African evergreen tree. Traditionally, pygeum has been used by African healers in the treatment of urinary disorders. An extract made from the bark should be taken at dosages of 100 mg once or twice a day, standardized to contain 14% triterpenes, including beta-sitosterol and

0.5% n-docosanal, for at least two months.

Studies have shown pygeum to reduce urinary symptoms associated with BPH[5]. Pygeum may be more effective than saw palmetto berry when prostate secretion is impaired—it has been shown to increase it. So pygeum may be an excellent herb when low sperm motility due to reduced prostatic secretion is the cause of the infertility. If you are suffering from BPH, pygeum can also help you to attain an erection. Pygeum and saw palmetto can be used very well together.

Nettle Root

Nettle root is another great herbal answer to BPH. Double-blind research has shown the root of the stinging nettle to be far better than a placebo, and it not only helps the symptoms, but actually significantly shrinks the prostate[6].

Other Help

Flower pollen, with its high quantity of plant flavonoids, has been shown to be effective in reducing symptoms of BPH[7]. In one study, 85% of the men who received a pollen extract showed improvement[8]. Other flavonoids may also prove useful.

The amino acids L-glutamic acid, L-alanine, and glycine may also shrink the prostrate and improve the symptoms of BPH[9]. Some have found them as effective as pollen.

Other possible treatments include various kinds of sitz baths in which the pelvic region is submerged in hot, cold, or tepid water for varying degrees of time. Sitz baths can be helpful since they tend to bring the blood into the abdominal region or move it away, helping to clear out obstructions.

Food and a Healthy Prostate

Equally important is that men with BPH (and everyone else who wishes to be healthy) avoid foods grown with pesticides, since pesticides have been shown to cause an increase in dihydrotestosterone in the prostate[10]. It is important that you avoid spraying your lawn and using chemicals in your home and at work. These can contribute to BPH. Also avoid storing food in plastics and consuming animal products, which can all increase the bad hormones that can contribute to BPH. Treatment and prevention of BPH involves a diet rich in whole foods that are free of toxins, chemicals, and pesticides. Especially important is a diet that is high in fibre to help rid the body of built-up toxins; a diet rich in chlorophyll and high in vitamins and minerals such as selenium, calcium, magnesium, germanium, zinc, flavonoids, and carotenes can help to rid the body of toxins[11]. Foods rich in vitamin C, E, choline, and inositol may also benefit the prostate gland. Soy foods also help to prevent BPH and even prostate cancer. Try taking kelp, which is rich in minerals and can help to supply crucial nutrients that may be missing from your diet. Kelp can also help to remove toxins from the body. Things to avoid are alcohol, especially beer, and stress, both of which can greatly increase the likelihood of developing BPH.

Anti-histamines can also aggravate BPH and long-term use may even contribute to its development.

TREATMENT SUMMARY

Diet & Lifestyle
- Eat half a cup of pumpkin seeds a day
- Eat a diet rich in essential fatty acids, fibre, chlorophyll, and soy
- Eat organic foods that are grown without pesticide
- Avoid animal products
- Avoid alcohol, especially beer

Nutritional Supplements
- Zinc: 50mg a day
- Copper: 2-3mg a day
- B6: 50mg one to two times a day

Herbs
- Saw palmetto berry: 320mg a day standardized for 85-95% fatty acids and sterols
- You can add one, or a combination, of:
  - Pygeum: 100mg of extract standardized for 14% triterpenes, including β-sitosterol and 0.05% n-docosanol

- Nettle root: 3-6g or 600-1,200mg 5:1 extract a day
- Flower pollen: 63-126mg two to three times a day

ENDNOTES

1. Fahim, M., *et al*. Zinc treatment for the reduction of hyperplasia of the prostrate. *Fed Proc* 1976; 35:361.

2. Klein, L. A., J. S. Stoff. Prostaglandins and the prostate: An hypothesis on the etiology of benign prostatic hyperplasia. *Prostate* 1983; 4:247–51.

3. Carraro, J. C., *et al*. Comparison of phytotherapy (Permixon®) with finasteride in the treatment of benign prostate hyperplasia: a randomized international study of 1,098 patients. *Prostate* 1996; 29:231–40; Wilt, T. J., *et al*. Saw palmetto extracts for treatment of benign prostatic hyperplasia. A systematic review. *JAMA* 1998; 280:1604–09; Debruyne, F., *et al*. Comparison of phytotherapeutic agent (Permixon) with an alpha-blocker (Tamsulosin) in the treatment of benign prostatic hyperplasia: A 1-year randomized international study. *European Urology* 2002; 41:497–506.

4. Champault, G., *et al*. The medical treatment of prostatic adenoma. A controlled study: PA-109 versus placebo in 110 patients. *Ann Urol* 1984; 18:407–10; Braeckman, J. The extract of Werenoa repens in the treatment of benign prostatic hyperplasia: A multicenter open study. *Curr Ther Res* 1994; 55:776–85; Bach, D., L. Ebeling. Long-term drug treatment of benign prostatic hyperplasia—results of a prospective 3-year multicenter study using *Sabal* extract IDS 89. *Phytomedicine* 1996; 3:105–11; Carraro, J.C., *et al*. Comparison of phytotherapy (Permixon®) with finasteride in the treatment of benign prostate hyperplasia: a randomized international study of 1,098 patients. *Prostate* 1996; 29:231–40; Wilt, T. J., *et al*. Saw palmetto extracts for treatment of benign prostatic hyperplasia. A systematic review. *JAMA* 1998; 280:1604–09; Debruyne, F., *et al*. Comparison of phytotherapeutic agent (Permixon) with an alpha-blocker (Tamsulosin) in the treatment of benign prostatic hyperplasia: A 1-year randomized international study. *European Urology* 2002; 41:497–506; Boyle, P., *et.al*. Updated meta-analysis of clinical trials of *Serenoa repens* extract in the treatment of symptomatic benign prostatic hyperplasia. *BJU International* 2004; 93:751.

5. Duvia, R., G. P. Radice, R. Galdini. Advances in the phytotherapy of prostatic hypertrophy. *Med Praxis* 1983; 4:143–48; Andro, M. C., J. P. Riffaud. *Pygeum africanum* extract for the treatment of patients with benign prostatic hyperplasia: a review of 25 years of published experience. *Curr Ther Res* 1995; 56:796–817; Ishani, A., *et al. Pygeum africanum* for the treatment of patients with benign prostatic hyperplasia: A systematic review and quantitative meta-analysis. *Am J Med* 2000; 109:654–64.

6. Safarineiead, M. R. Urtica dioica for treatment of benign prostatic hyperplasia: a prospective, randomized, double-blind, placebo-controlled, cross-over study. *J Herb Pharmacother* 2005; 5:1–11.

7. Buck, A. C., *et al.* Treatment of outflow tract obstruction due to benign prostatic hyperplasia with the pollen extract, cernilton. A double-blind, placebo-controlled study. *Br J Urol* 1990; 66:398–404; Becker, H., L. Ebeling. Conservative therapy of benign prostatic hyperplasia (BPH) with Cernilton. *Urologe (B)* 1988; 28:301–06.

8. Yasumoto, R. *et al.* Clinical evaluation of long-term treatment using Cernilton pollen extract in patients with benign prostatic hyperplasia. *Clinical Therapeutics* 1995; 17:82–86.

9. Feinblatt, H. M., *et al.* Palliative treatment of benign prostatic hypertrophy: Value of glycine, alanine, glutamic acid combination. *J Maine Med Assoc* 1958; 46:99–102; Dumrau, F. Benign prostatic hyperplasia: Amino acid therapy for symptomatic relief. *Am J Geriatr* 1962; 10:426–30.

10. Ask-Upmark, E. Prostatitis and its treatment. *Acta Med Scan* 1967; 181:355–57; Kappas, A., *et al.* Nutrition-endocrine interactions. Induction of reciprocal changes in the delta-5-alpha-reduction of testosterone and the cytochrome P-450-dependent oxidation of estradiol by dietary macronutrients in men. *Proct Natl Acad Sci USA* 1983; 80:7646–49.

11. Murray, M. T., J. Pizzorno. *Encyclopedia of Natural Medicine.* Rocklin, CA: Prima, (1991), p.483.

Chapter Eleven

FLY ON THE WALL: SEX QUESTIONS COMMONLY ASKED IN LINDA'S CLINIC

What can I do to make sex less painful, or even possible? I have been unable to tolerate, or even achieve, penetration.

This problem occurs frequently with young women who may be having sex for the first time, small women, women who have not had sex for a while, women in menopause who are vaginally dry, and women who may have some kind of problem such as scar tissue, infection, or endometriosis. In general, here are some healthy, easy tips to help sex be less painful. It is important to stretch out the vaginal cavity, so, while in the shower, use your fingers to gently stretch out the vaginal cavity daily for a while until improvement happens. Also, consider getting on top during sex: this position makes guiding the penis in easier and less painful as the woman can control it. Ask the man to go slowly and gently until penetration is achieved. Also, massage the muscles between the vagina and the anus, relax them and breathe deeply: this helps to make penetration easier. Using lubrication can help: some good ones are topical vitamin E oil or even olive oil or almond oil. Be careful, though, when using a condom because oil-based products may compromise them. Vitamin E especially helps menopausal women who are vaginally dry. If infection is present, treat it; if endometriosis is present, treat it (see our book, *The Family Naturopathic Encyclopedia*). Structural problems often require further aid. Also, taking relaxing herbs such as skullcap, kava kava, chamomile, valerian, lemon balm, oats, passionflower, and catnip can help.

I ejaculate too soon. What can I do?

This is probably the most common of all the male sexual problems. Ejaculating prematurely is often due to hormonal imbalances and weak kidney energy, according to Chinese medicine. Sometimes herbs that strengthen the kidneys help, for instance, eleuthero (formerly Siberian ginseng), ho shou wu, astragalus, nettle, ginger, or rehmannia. It is a good idea to get a program tailored to your body's own individual needs. Also, taking relaxing herbs such as hops, skullcap, kava kava, chamomile, valerian, lemon balm, oats, passionflower, and catnip can help. Hops is used for men with excessive sexual desire. Also calcium, magnesium, B vitamins, and adrenal-supporting herbs like licorice, ginseng, rhodiola, suma, and ashwagandha can help. Rhoidola rosea has been show to help specifically with this problem (see erectile dysfunction chapter). Saw palmetto can also help to correct hormone issues. Getting the man to focus on some nonsexual image during sex, and gently squeezing the penis tip—some say base—or pulling the testicles away from the body can help to hold off ejaculation. Look up the start-stop exercise technique developed in the 1950's by Dr. James Semans (how do these things happen?). Most of the premature ejaculation programs used today by sex therapists are based on it.

The woman does not achieve orgasm. What can we do?

There can be many reasons for this problem. One is poor nutrition, so eat well and take a high-potency multivitamin/mineral formula. Other reasons include hormone and endocrine imbalances. Chastetree berry, wild yam, black cohosh, red clover, natural progesterone cream, fennel, licorice, soy, ginseng, and dong quai may help by balancing hormones or positively affecting reproductive health. They can bring up low progesterone and estrogen levels. Relaxant herbs such as skullcap, kava kava, valerian, oats, passionflower, lemon balm, chamomile, and catnip may help if the problem is due to nerves, stress, or psychological exhaustion. Suma, ashwagandha, licorice, and ginseng may help if the problem is due to nervous exhaustion or weakness. Damiana and/or muira puama may help. Poor blood-flow problems or the side effects of some antidepressants may respond to *Ginkgo biloba*. The same remedies apply to men. Structural problems and other deeper issues need to be individually addressed. Also, consider that many women do not easily have an orgasm from penetration, so manual stimulation or oral stimulation of the clitoris can help greatly.

After sex the woman frequently reports burning or pain. What can we do?

This discomfort can be due to irritation, candida, or infection, among other possibilities. Always find out first what it is. After sex, wash the area with a dilute mixture of tea tree oil and water, or goldenseal and water, front to back. Also, insert probiotics vaginally and allow to dissolve. This step will usually help prevent and treat infection and candida. Take probiotics orally as well as goldenseal and/or other antibiotic herbs and/or anti-candida agents. In other words, treat for candida and infection if present (see the candida and urinary tract infection chapters). Taking cranberry after sex has been shown in double-blind research to prevent infection. These solutions can sometimes help even if no infection or candida is obviously present. Also, try applying an aloe vera lip balm to the outside affected area or try vitamin E oil or a slippery elm poultice for irritation and pain. Soaking in a salt-water sitz bath can also be useful.

Sometimes I bleed vaginally after intercourse. What can I do?

The reason for bleeding should first be addressed, and if no obvious problem is present, then it is often due to irritation or to causing old, stagnant blood to flow. Try packing the area with an astringent poultice made from comfrey, raspberry leaf, or yarrow. Yarrow, nettle, and/or raspberry leaf can also be taken orally to stop bleeding. Dong quai, taken daily internally may help if the problem is due to old stagnant blood.

I am vaginally dry. What can I do to make sex less painful?

Although this question is covered above, a more thorough answer is given here. Vaginal dryness is often due to low hormone levels or out-of-balance hormones. So first, see the chapter on menopause: this information will also apply to women who have no periods or miss a lot of periods due to low or imbalanced hormones. You may want to try taking one or more of the following: black cohosh, licorice, red clover, chastetree berry, vitamin E, vitamin C, and bioflavonoids or soy. Also, try inserting vitamin-E-oil capsules vaginally, or use vitamin-E oil topically. Aloe vera lip balm is also good topically. Probiotics inserted vaginally may also help. Women who miss their periods altogether may benefit from taking rhodiola, which can normalize this problem and also correct related issues.

I cannot ejaculate, although I can achieve and maintain an erection. What can I do?

First, rule out structural or other medical conditions. If no obvious cause is found, your problem may be due to low adrenal function from stress and/ or exhaustion. Try any of ginseng, rhodiola, suma, licorice, or ashwagandha. Poor nutrition may be playing a role, so follow the dietary suggestions given in the book and take a high-potency multivitamin/ mineral formula. Also useful may be *Ginkgo biloba*, damiana, and muira puama.

I cannot maintain and/or get an erection. What can I do?

First, determine the cause and rule out structural or other problems. Next, refer to the chapter on erectile dysfunction. You may want to try using one of many herbs—muira puama, damiana, ginseng, *Ginkgo biloba*, horny goat weed, saw palmetto, suma, ashwagandha, licorice, or rhodiola. Also try B-vitamins, arginine, vitamin C, vitamin E, zinc, and cholesterol-lowering herbs and nutrients if atherosclerosis is present.

My penis is sore after sex. What can I do?

First, make sure it is not from a sexually transmitted disease or other infection. If it is, treat it. If no cause is found, it can be due to friction and/or irritation. You can try bathing in a salt-water sitz bath and/or try applying aloe vera gel/balm or vitamin-E oil topically. Also, try a poultice made of slippery elm powder topically. For inflamed penises, or even local infections, try a powder, applied topically, of slippery elm powder, marshmallow-root powder, and goldenseal powder. Herbalist Rosemary Gladstar says she has found this solution to be quick and effective. Or try a strong tea made of goldenseal and comfrey and soak the penis in it, like a sitz bath. Treat internally, too, with goldenseal, Echinacea, wild indigo, garlic, licorice, and/or other immune herbs. Also, try topical decoctions of witch hazel bark, white oak bark, and raspberry leaf. Candida may be present, so check for that and treat if needed.

Tip: Try doing Kegel exercises. They strengthen the genito-urinary system, which not only helps with bladder control, but also enhances sexual performance, increases circulation to the pelvis, and increases the overall health of the reproductive area. This is true for both men and women. To do the exercise, squeeze the pubococcygeal muscle, a large band-like muscle that runs from the pubic bone to the coccyx. It's the muscle you feel when you tighten your anus. If you squeeze it, it can stop urine in mid flow. To do Kegels, pull inward and upward while tightening the anus at the same time. Pull up as hard as you can, hold, relax, and release. Repeat ten to a hundred times per day. Rosemary Gladstar says that it is guaranteed to make your sex life better, especially if your partner is doing them, too.

Appendix

WHAT YOU CAN DO TO HAVE A HEALTHY REPRODUCTIVE SYSTEM

The Do's and Don'ts of Diet and Lifestyle

- Increase essential unsaturated oils
- Eliminate trans fatty acids
- Increase vegetable protein
- Decrease animal protein
- Decrease dairy consumption: dairy products and other animal products contain substances that raise estrogen, leading to infertility. As dairy consumption goes up, the more males become infertile. Avoidance of hormone-fed animal products and dairy products are a must for men with low sperm counts or low testosterone.
- Increase whole grains and complex carbohydrates
- Decrease refined carbohydrates
- Get lots of iron from fruits, veggies, beans, and supplements, but not from red meat
- Drink water, not sugary soft drinks
- Lose weight if you're overweight

- If you're underweight from over-exercising and under-eating, work to correct the issues and correct the problem
- Exercise
- Don't smoke
- Don't use caffeine
- Avoid chemicals and food additives: many environmental toxins contain estrogen that damages male fertility. Avoid such chemicals as DDT, PCBs, and dioxin found in the environment. Even though DDT has been banned, it stays in the soil for twenty years or more, so it is still found in the soil and in the food that is grown in that soil.
- Avoid storing food in plastics
- Avoid pesticides
- Avoid exposure to radiation
- Avoid certain prescription drugs
- Avoid exposure to drinking water with estrogen in it: this means water stored in certain plastic bottles. Also, water-treatment plants allow excreted synthetic estrogens, perhaps from birth control pills, to get into our drinking water. So use water that has been purified or is in safe containers like glass or BPA-free plastics.
- If your testosterone is low or your estrogen is high, eat soy products and other legumes: these foods are phytoestrogenic and can work to lower high estrogen levels in the body by stealing receptor sites from your body's own stronger estrogen. In women with low estrogen, they can actually raise it, by adding a small bit of estrogen to your body's depleted estrogen. So they are also vital for female fertility. Their testosterone-like phytosterols may also be used by your body to produce needed hormones.

All of these factors have been shown to increase your chances of getting pregnant. And, of course, these recommendations are exactly the diet that our modern culture has moved away from.

The Ideal Diet for a Healthy Reproductive System
- at least 6 to 9 servings of vegetables a day, from a wide variety of colours and types of vegetables. Include at least one deep green leafy veggie a

day, and eat sea vegetables frequently: they are high in iodine and help to support the thyroid glands.

- at least 2 to 4 servings a day of fruit
- at least 3 to 6 servings a day of whole grains
- 1 to 3 servings a day of legumes
- a handful of raw, unsalted seeds and nuts
- 1 to 3 tablespoons of milled flax seeds or uncooked flax-seed oil
- use first-cold-pressed extra virgin olive oil to cook with
- drink 8 glasses of water a day away from meals
- try to eat at least some of your food raw

Index